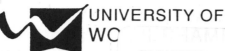
Rheuma...

J

C... ...ysician in
R... ...logy, Nether Edge Hospital,
S... ...l; Head, Sheffield Centre for
R... ...umatic Diseases; Honorary
Clinical Lecturer in Rheumatic
Diseases, University of Sheffield

Churchill Livingstone

EDINBURGH LON... ...AND TOKYO 1992

In general, rheumatology is a specialty eminently suited to pictorial representation. Surface colour changes and alterations in the morphology of the limbs and trunk combine to form a myriad of unique clinical patterns. Once seen, these are rarely forgotten.

The source of this collection is largely personal and was started almost 30 years ago when the author was a house physician. Here and there, however, it has been necessary to take advantage of the kind cooperation of the following colleagues to provide slides of rarities or simply to fill gaps created by lost or unrecognized clinical opportunity: Dr R. S. Amos, Dr N. A. Barrington, Dr D. E. Bax, Dr M. J. Brown, Dr G. N. Chandler, Dr D. Cumberland, Dr M. S. Derini, Mr R. A. Elson, the late Dr H. G. Garland, Professor F. D. Hart, Dr P. Hughes, Dr G. R. Newns, Dr N. R. Rowell, Professor R. G. G. Russell, the late Dr R. N. Tattersall, Dr J. Winfield, Professor V. Wright.

I also wish to thank my secretary, Mrs Pat Drake, for typing the manuscript and the publishers for guidance in its presentation.

Sheffield   J. M. H. M.

Contents

1 / Rheumatoid arthritis (RA)

Definition   Chronic polyarthritis characterized by bilateral symmetrical joint disease, radiological erosions, positive tests for rheumatoid factor and, pathologically, a chronic proliferative synovitis with villous hypertrophy, infiltration by lymphocytes and plasma cells and by nodules. It is a multisystem disorder, justifying the use by some of the term 'rheumatoid *disease*'. The condition is often included under the systemic connective tissue diseases (collagenoses). Diagnostic criteria are available.

Prevalence   RA affects 6% of females and 2% of males and has a world-wide distribution. It is the most common inflammatory disease of joints in UK (affecting about 1.5×10^6) and elsewhere. Onset: 16–70 yr; most often: 20–55 yr.

Aetiology   The cause is unknown. A prominent feature is the formation of immune complexes within the joint. These activate complement and attract neutrophils. Phagocytosis of immune complexes by neutrophils leads to release of chemical mediators of inflammation. Continued inflammation stimulates the formation of a proliferative synovitis. This hypertrophic granulation tissue is called pannus (Fig. 1). It is this that is responsible for causing joint erosions. These can be seen clearly as macroscopic lesions on the joint surface (Fig. 1) or on X-ray (Fig. 2).

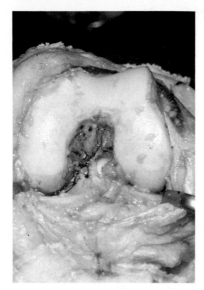

Fig. 1 RA. Synovial hypertrophy and erosions of articular cartilage.

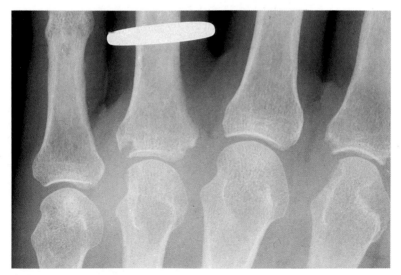

Fig. 2 RA. Periarticular erosions of MCP joints.

Clinical features   **Joint disease**

Hands. A typical onset is the appearance of pain, stiffness (usually early morning stiffness), swelling and tenderness of the knuckle joints—proximal interphalangeal (PIPs) and metacarpophalangeal (MCPs). Fusiform swelling of the PIP joints gives the fingers a characteristic spindle shape, and the knuckles (PIPs and MCPs) may show dusky discoloration or pigmentation. (Fig. 3). With more advanced disease, MCP subluxation and ulnar deviation of the fingers occur (Fig. 4), and also 'boutonnière' and 'swan-neck' deformities (Fig. 5). The wrists are also often involved. This feature, together with the absence of distal interphalangeal (DIP) involvement with Heberden's nodes, helps to differentiate rheumatoid arthritis (RA) of the hands from that other common arthropathy—osteoarthrosis (OA). If Bouchard's nodes (OA of PIP joints) are present they are differentiated as hard swellings, compared with the softer joint swelling in rheumatoid arthritis. However, as both are common diseases they may co-exist. Psoriatic arthritis will usually be obvious because of the asymmetry and oligoarticular pattern of involvement, apart from the presence of skin and/or nail involvement. Gout barely comes into the differential diagnosis as it causes severe inflammatory features, and in some patients tophi will make the diagnosis clear. Carcinoma arthritis may be indistinguishable from rheumatoid arthritis.

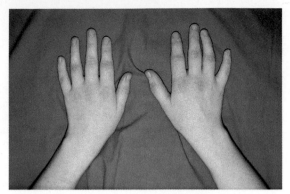

Fig. 3 Early RA. Discoloration over PIPs and MCPs, and slight 'spindling'.

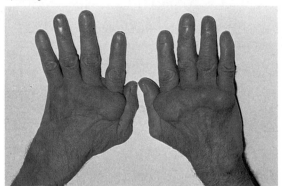

Fig. 4 RA at later stage. Considerable MCP joint thickening, subluxation and ulnar deviation.

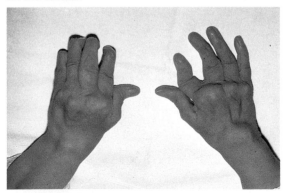

Fig. 5 Advanced RA. 'Swan-neck' deformities and synovial thickening of wrists.

Clinical features (contd)

Feet. Irritable MTP joints are the main source of trouble. Patients feel as though there are pebbles in their shoe. On examination calluses may be seen over these joints (Fig. 6), and the counterpart deformities to those seen in the hand may be obvious (Figs 6 & 7)—fibular deviation of the toes. Other features may be present including discharging fistulae (Fig. 8).

Other joints. Progression of the disease may result in spread to almost all peripheral joints. The spine (limited to the upper cervical region) may be involved. Although less common, even the arytenoid joints (synovial joints) may become affected.

Soft-tissue rheumatic manifestations

Bursal swellings and rupture. An important complication is the enlargement and rupture of bursal cysts near joints. Notable is popliteal (Baker's) cyst rupture causing leakage of synovial fluid from the knee into the calf. This may be diagnosed erroneously as a deep vein thrombosis. In the patient shown in Fig. 9 the cyst had become infected.

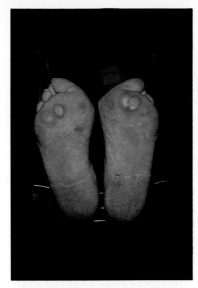

Fig. 6 RA. Calluses over subluxated MTP joints and fibular deviation of toes.

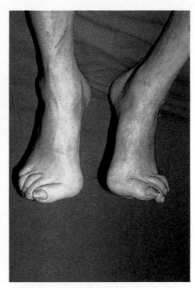

Fig. 7 RA. Marked hallux valgus and fibular deviation of other toes.

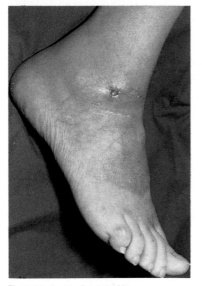

Fig. 8 RA. Healing fistula had been discharging synovial fluid from ankle joint.

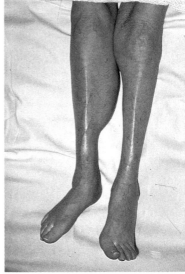

Fig. 9 RA. Ruptured Baker's cyst with massive calf extension containing pus.

Clinical features
(contd)

Diseases of tendons and tendon sheaths:

- *Rupture of an extensor tendon or tendons* may occur due to the destructive effect of synovial proliferation and roughened bones on the dorsum of the wrist. Extensor tendon rupture manifests as a 'dropped finger' with inability to extend the digit, and there is usually prominent synovial thickening on the dorsum of the wrist (Fig. 10). This diagnosis is important, as splintage to encourage natural union or surgical repair is often beneficial.
- *Rupture of a flexor tendon or tendons* may occur due to the same effect on the palmar aspect of the wrist. This presents as an inability to bend the finger. Prominent synovial bulging is usually also evident on the front of the wrist (Fig. 11).
- *Trigger finger* may occur due to tendon sheath involvement when the patient is unable to straighten the finger spontaneously (Fig. 12). A tendon or tendon sheath nodule may be palpable in the affected area.

Tendon or tendon sheath complications and associated deformities should not be confused with finger deformities due to interphalangeal (IP) joint disease (Fig. 13).

Nerve entrapment syndromes. Most common is the carpal tunnel syndrome which may occur at any stage in rheumatoid arthritis (see p. 91).

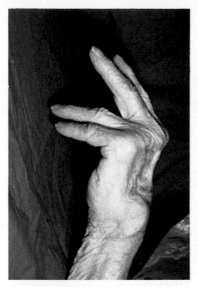

Fig. 10 RA. Extensor tendon rupture. Note swelling on back of wrist.

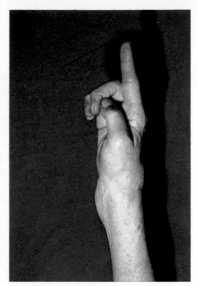

Fig. 11 RA. Flexor tendon rupture. Note swelling on front of wrist.

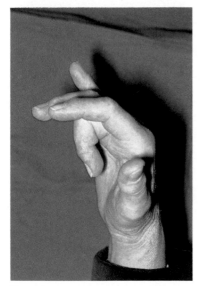

Fig. 12 RA. 'Trigger finger' due to tendon sheath nodule.

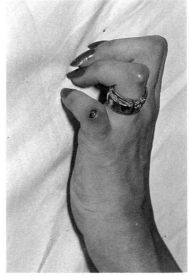

Fig. 13 RA. Clawed fingers due to rapidly progressive arthritis of PIP joints.

Clinical features
(contd)

Systemic manifestations

General. These include weight loss, low-grade fever, lymph node enlargement, oedema, anaemia, osteoporosis (and fractures), infections and amyloidosis.

Arteritis. This is an indication of severe disease. In the fingers it gives rise to nail-fold infarcts—small brown/black marks (Fig. 14) which are often unnoticed by the patient. These may also occur elsewhere on the fingers (Fig. 15). More extensive arteritis is manifest by more obvious lesions, and even by extensive areas of gangrene (Fig. 16). In this instance, after the gangrenous finger tips had sloughed, they 'regenerated' (including reformation of the nail), although the fingers were shorter than before. Infarcts may also occur in relation to rheumatoid nodules (see p. 11); a typical example is shown in Figure 17.

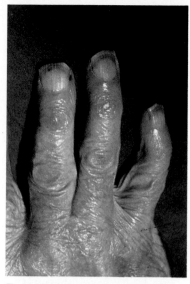

Fig. 14 RA. Nail fold, nail bed and dermal infarcts. (White nails incidental.)

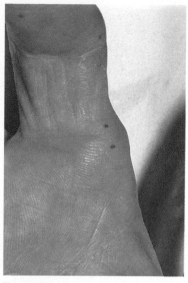

Fig. 15 RA. Dermal infarcts (resembling small pigmented naevi).

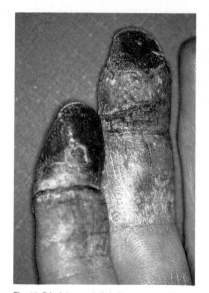

Fig. 16 RA. Advanced digital gangrene with demarcation lines.

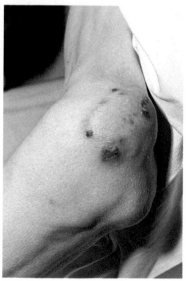

Fig. 17 RA. Dermal infarcts overlying elbow nodules.

Clinical features
(contd)

Subcutaneous nodules. These are painless fleshy lumps varying from the size of a pea to that of a tangerine (0.5–3 cm diameter). They are found typically over the olecranon (Figs 18 & 19), but may also be found over other bony prominences (e.g. bridge of nose, occiput, sacrum) or arising from tendons (particularly the tendo Achilles). They may also occur more 'deeply', and their appearance in the lungs (in patients with pneumoconiosis) is termed Caplan's syndrome (Fig. 20). Rheumatoid nodules only occur in patients with positive tests for rheumatoid factor (often highly positive) and are virtually diagnostic of the disorder.

Myelopathy and neuropathy. Although caused by different mechanisms, these neurological complications may be included here. Severe arthritis of the mid and upper cervical spine may cause damage to the cervical cord, presenting as tetraparesis or even tetraplegia. The spinal arthritis is usually considerable and associated with subluxation (Fig. 21). Neuropathy, either mononeuritis multiplex or polyneuropathy, is another neurological manifestation of severe systemic rheumatoid arthritis.

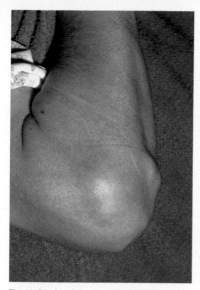

Fig. 18 RA. Small/medium sized elbow nodules.

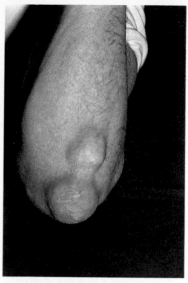

Fig. 19 RA. Large nodules over distal ulna and in olecranon bursa.

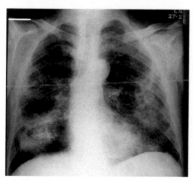

Fig. 20 Caplan's syndrome. Massive rheumatoid nodules in both pneumoconiotic lung fields.

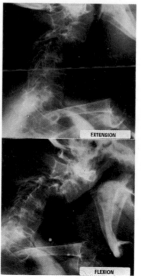

Fig. 21 RA. Severe mid-cervical spondylopathy with inter-vertebral subluxation anteriorly.

Clinical features
(contd)

Eye disease. Several ocular manifestations are seen in this type of arthritis. The most common is episcleritis (Fig. 22). This is usually asymptomatic. More serious is scleritis (Fig. 22). The gravest ocular complication is scleromalacia perforans. This results in immediate and permanent blindness.

Other 'systemic' manifestations. Ulceration of the skin, usually over the sacrum (Fig. 23) or on the legs, is due to large-vessel arteritis. Another surface feature is palmar erythema (Fig. 24), and it is important not to assume liver disease from this sign in rheumatoid patients. Other systemic features are mentioned under the related syndromes (Sjögren's syndrome, p. 15; Felty's syndrome, p. 17).

Radiological
features

Early: juxta-articular osteoporosis and erosions (see Fig. 2, p. 2).

Late: loss of joint space, bone destruction and subluxation (see Fig. 21, p. 12).

Laboratory
features

Anaemia and raised ESR are present in active disease. Positive tests are seen for rheumatoid factor (e.g. latex, Rose–Waaler). ANF is often positive, and LE cells are present in 10%. Anti-DNA antibodies are not present, while HLA Dw4 and HLA DRw4 are present in over 50%. Synovial fluid: turbid, yellow/green, low viscosity, clot-positive, approximately 30 000 WBC ($\times$ 10^9/dl)—all characteristics of a 'non-specific' inflammatory exudate. (Gout and pseudogout fluids contain crystals, and the fluid of septic arthritis is culture-positive.)

Management

Involves advice/instruction; drugs: non-steroidal anti-inflammatory drugs at first—supplement, if necessary, with small-dose corticosteroids and/or a remission-inducing agent (e.g. gold, penicillamine or antimalarials); rest; exercises; aids and appliances; surgery.

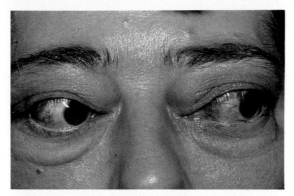

Fig. 22 RA. Episcleritis in the right eye; episcleritis and scleritis in the left eye.

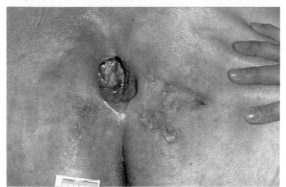

Fig. 23 RA. Deep ulcer surrounded by healing ulcers.

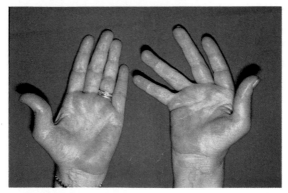

Fig. 24 RA. Palmar erythema.

2 / Sjögren's syndrome

Definition Sjögren's syndrome (after Henrick S. C. Sjögren, born 1899) is a triad of defective lacrimal secretion (keratoconjunctivitis sicca), defective salivary secretion (xerostomia) and a systemic connective tissue disorder. The term sicca syndrome is applied when the only features are dry eyes and mouth.

Prevalence Most often seen in rheumatoid arthritis, 30% of whom show features of the syndrome. F:M = 9:1.

Aetiology Immunological and immunogenetic factors have been reported. There may be more than one aetiological type.

Clinical features **Eyes**
Gritty irritation and redness, with early morning stickiness, and reduction in tear secretion (often not noticed by the patient) are the usual features. The dryness may lead to conjunctivitis (Fig. 25), keratitis, corneal erosions and even vascularization of the cornea.

GI tract
The salivary glands are usually normal in size but may be enlarged (Fig. 26). Diminished salivary flow is associated with dryness, smoothness and increased sensitivity of the lips and tongue, and dental caries are accelerated (Fig. 27).

Other features
These include respiratory infections, renal tubular defects, atrophic vaginitis and lymphomata.

Laboratory features Diagnosis is established by positive Schirmer's test (measurement of tear secretion with filter paper strip). Rose Bengal and slit lamp examinations are used to reveal corneal disease. Biopsy of salivary or lacrimal glands may be necessary to exclude sarcoidosis or malignancy.

Management ***Mouth:*** glycerine mouth wash and sucking lemon sweets.
Eyes: protection and instillation of artifical tears.

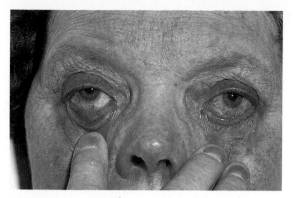

Fig. 25 Sjögren's syndrome. Bilateral conjunctivitis in a patient with dry eyes.

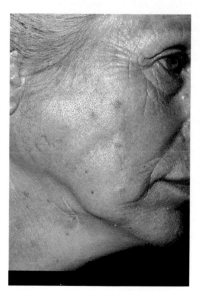

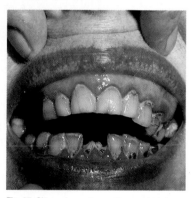

Fig. 27 Sjögren's syndrome. Severe dental caries and gingivitis.

Fig. 26 Sjögren's syndrome. Parotid gland hypertrophy. Note scars from duct surgery and biopsy.

3 / Felty's syndrome

Definition A syndrome comprising chronic arthritis, splenomegaly and granulocytopenia, in which the lymphoreticular features of rheumatoid arthritis assume an exaggerated form. It is named after A. R. Felty (born 1895).

Prevalence The precise prevalence is not known. It affects about 1% of patients with rheumatoid arthritis. Splenomegaly alone is more common (about 6.5%). F:M = 2:1. Onset occurs after at least 10 yr of rheumatoid arthritis. Usual age of onset: 50–70 yr.

Aetiology Variant of seropositive rheumatoid arthritis.

Clinical features
- Severe joint disease (Fig. 28).
- Splenomegaly (Fig. 28). This is often massive.
- Hepatomegaly (Fig. 28). This is usually slight.
- Leg ulcers (Fig. 29).
- Pigmentation—especially legs (Fig. 29).
- Increased susceptibility to infection.

Radiological features Same as in rheumatoid arthritis, with severe destructive arthritis. Abdominal X-ray may reveal splenomegaly.

Laboratory features These include relative and absolute granulocytopenia, mild to moderate anaemia (most patients), thrombocytopenia (38%), positive rheumatoid factor (98%), positive ANF and LE cells. Anti-DNA is not raised.

Management Aim to reverse haematological abnormalities.
- Splenectomy may be indicated if significant morbidity.
- Drugs have been tried: include corticosteroids, gold, penicillamine, high-dose testosterone (but not for females) and lithium salts.

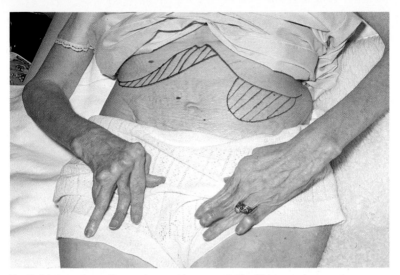

Fig. 28 Felty's syndrome. Severe, rheumatoid-pattern arthritis with hepatosplenomegaly.

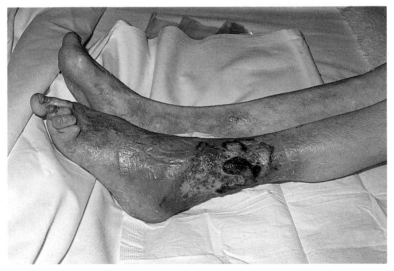

Fig. 29 Felty's syndrome. Severe leg ulcers with pigmentation. Note also arthritis of feet.

4 / Ankylosing spondylitis

Definition A chronic inflammatory disease of the spine and sacroiliac joints causing progressive restriction of spinal movement. It is associated with radiological calcification of spinal ligaments.

Synonyms Spondylitis ankylopoetica, spondylitis rhizomélique, von Bechterew's disease and morbus Bechterew–Marie–Strümpell.

Prevalence Established disease: approximately 0.1%. M:F = 5:1. Age of onset is usually 15–30 yr. The disease is less common in American Negroes, and more common in American Indians, than in Caucasians.

Aetiology Probably due to a combination of genetic and environmental factors. Genetic transmission is not clear and both Mendelian dominant and multifactorial mechanisms have been reported. Environmental factors could involve infective agents (e.g. *Klebsiella*) and other factors such as trauma.

Clinical features **Spine**
- Pain—worsening at night, and stiffness most noticeable in the morning on wakening.
- Postural changes may be noted by patient, or only brought to their attention by others. These characteristically involve rounding of the shoulders and slight dorsal kyphosis—the 'hang-dog posture' seen early on (Fig. 30). Later the stoop may become more pronounced (Fig. 31), and in extreme cases will limit forward vision.
- Spinal motion in forward flexion (Fig. 32) and in other directions becomes limited, as does chest expansion.

Peripheral joints
The 'root' joints (hips and shoulders) are most commonly affected (40%). Of other peripheral joints, the knees are most often involved (Fig. 33).

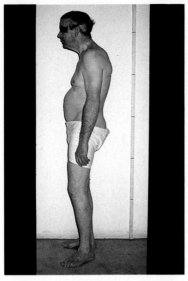

Fig. 30 Ankylosing spondylitis. Early postural changes—the 'hang-dog posture'.

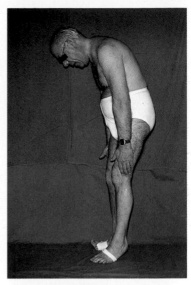

Fig. 31 Ankylosing spondylitis. Advanced stoop with limited forward vision.

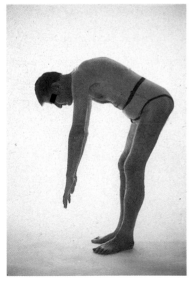

Fig. 32 Ankylosing spondylitis. Limited spinal flexion (in patient asked to touch toes).

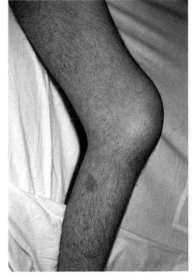

Fig. 33 Ankylosing spondylitis. Active arthritis of knee with wasted quadriceps.

Radiological
features

Pelvis
The crucial radiological feature is sacroiliitis, the presence of which is a *sine qua non* for diagnosing the disease by international agreement. The components of radiological sacroiliitis are:

- sclerosis of the margins of the sacroiliac joint
- blurring of the joint outline due to sacral and iliac erosions
- narrowing and eventually fusion (ankylosis).

The pelvic X-ray is invaluable as, in addition to showing sacroiliac arthritis (Fig. 34), it may show other features such as symphyseal arthritis, ischial and iliac exostoses, and hip arthritis.

Spine
The most characteristic lesion is the syndesmophyte, the basis of bony bridging. Figure 35 shows the various stages in the development of intervertebral ankylosis. Other characteristic spinal changes include: vertebral 'squaring', erosion of anterior vertebral corners (Romanus lesions) and disc calcification/ossification. Any region of the spine may be affected, but the thoracolumbar junction is the best place to look for early changes.

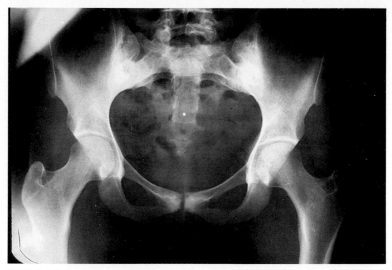

Fig. 34 Ankylosing spondylitis. Bilateral sacroiliitis and symphyseal arthritis.

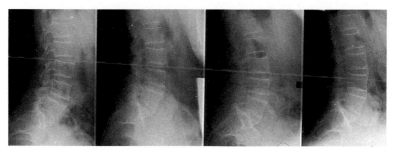

Fig. 35 Ankylosing spondylitis. Various stages of intervertebral ankylosis by syndesmophytes.

Co-diseases
- Iritis (25%)—often unilateral (Fig. 36).
- Aortic incompetence (1%) (Fig. 37) and, more commonly, cardiac conduction defects.

Less commonly:

- Cauda equina syndrome (Fig. 38).
- Atlantoaxial subluxation or spinal fracture.
- Apical pulmonary fibrosis (resembling tuberculosis).
- Amyloidosis.

Whether classed as co-diseases, complications, or 'overlap' features, patients with spondylitis may display manifestations characteristic of other spondarthritides: psoriasis, chronic inflammatory bowel disorders and genitourinary disease.

Laboratory features
ESR is raised in 80%, but may be normal even in quite active disease. Often mild anaemia is present. Test for rheumatoid factor is negative, and HLA B27 is present in 96%.

Management
- Analgesic/anti-inflammatory drugs (phenylbutazone and indomethacin are particularly helpful).
- Exercises to maintain mobility and prevent development of poor posture.
- Steroid injection of peripheral joints.
- Surgery. Hip replacement is most often indicated. Only rarely is spinal osteotomy needed, and even then only in special centres.
- Radiotherapy is becoming obsolete because of the risk of post-radiation malignancy.

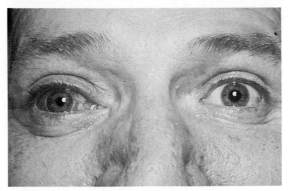

Fig. 36 Ankylosing spondylitis. Unilateral acute anterior uveitis (iritis).

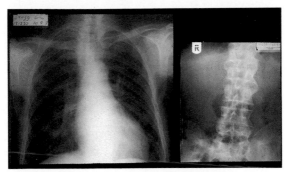

Fig. 37 Ankylosing spondylitis. Cardiomegaly due to aortic incompetence (*left*). Typical 'bamboo spine' in this patient (*right*).

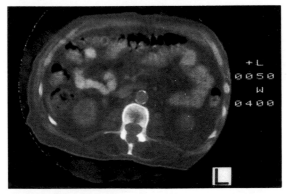

Fig. 38 Ankylosing spondylitis. Cauda equina lesion. Note erosions around spinal canal.

5 / **Psoriatic arthritis**

Definition   The association of skin or nail psoriasis with seronegative arthritis affecting peripheral and/or spinal joints.

Prevalence   Psoriasis affects 1–2% of the population. About 7% of psoriatics develop arthritis. Of these about 30% have sacroiliitis. M:F = 1:1 for psoriatic arthritis (about the same as in uncomplicated psoriasis—compare female preponderance in rheumatoid arthritis).

Aetiology   The condition is probably due to a combination of genetic and environmental factors. Heredity is probably non-Mendelian. Environmental factors could be multifactorial, including physical and emotional trauma, and infection.

Clinical features   **Dermatological manifestations**

Skin. The typical rash consists of salmon-pink, scaly plaques on extensor surfaces (Fig. 39), variants of this causing circinate, guttate or even exfoliative patterns. Of importance is the fact that lesions may be minimal (consisting of only a single spot a few millimetres in diameter) or 'hidden'. The scalp is a favourite location for hidden lesions (Fig. 40), but they may be found under the breasts, in the natal cleft or in the umbilicus.

Nail. Nail dystrophy affects about 80% with the uncomplicated skin condition. Typical changes include pitting (Fig. 41), onycholysis (Fig. 42) and other features such as horizontal ridging, keratosis or discoloration.

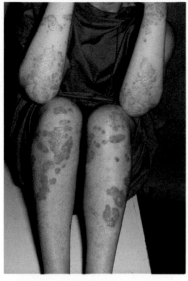

Fig. 39 Psoriatic arthritis. Typical rash (psoriasis vulgaris).

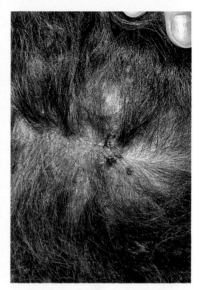

Fig. 40 Psoriatic arthritis. Patch of scalp psoriasis hidden by hair.

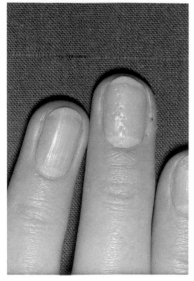

Fig. 41 Psoriatic arthritis. Nail pitting.

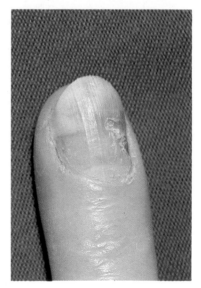

Fig. 42 Psoriatic arthritis. Onycholysis.

Clinical features
(contd)

Rheumatological manifestations

- The commonest pattern is an asymmetrical oligoarticular arthritis involving scattered knuckle joints—DIPs, PIPs or MCPs. A typical example is shown in Fig. 43. The mildness of this pattern of arthritis may lead to the diagnosis being overlooked.
- It may appear almost indistinguishable from rheumatoid arthritis.
- The 'textbook' pattern, less common than the above manifestations, is widespread involvement of DIP joints. Although characteristic, it has been over-emphasized in the past as it is seen in only about 5% of patients with psoriatic arthritis.
- 'Sausage digits'. They may affect the hands (Fig. 44) or feet (Fig. 45), and may be generalized involving all digits, or localized to one finger or toe. This appearance is due to combined IP arthritis and flexor tenosynovitis.
- Arthritis mutilans occurs rarely. This may be largely *erosive*, giving rise to 'opera-glass fingers' ('doigts-en-lorgnettes'), or *ankylosing*, giving rise to a rigid, clawed hand.
- Ankylosing spondylitis (see p. 29).

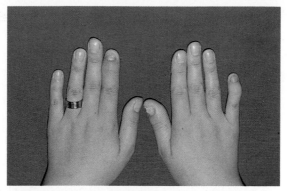

Fig. 43 Psoriatic arthritis. Typical asymmetrical oligoarticular involvement. Note nail dystrophy.

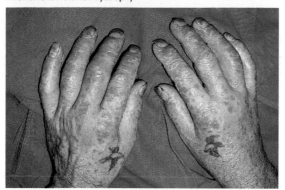

Fig. 44 Psoriatic arthritis. Severe arthropathy with 'sausage fingers'. Note nail dystrophy.

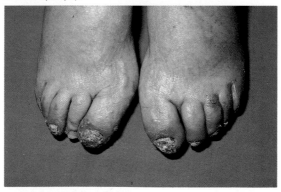

Fig. 45 Psoriatic arthritis. 'Sausage toes' and early toe deformities. Note nail dystrophy.

Radiological features

Often these are no more than periarticular soft-tissue swelling, small periarticular erosions or diminution of joint space with minimal or no deformity. Other less common radiological features, some of which are shown in Fig. 46, include:

- Erosion of terminal phalangeal tufts (acro-osteolysis).
- 'Whittling' of phalanges, metacarpals, and metatarsals.
- 'Cupping' of the proximal ends of phalanges. The combination of 'whittling' and 'cupping' may give rise to the 'pencil-in-cup deformity' or 'mushrooming'.
- Ankylosis of phalanges, metacarpals, and metatarsals.
- Severe destruction of isolated small joints.
- Predilection for DIP and PIP joints with relative sparing of MP joints (cf. rheumatoid arthritis).
- Tendency to involve the feet before the hands, as in Reiter's disease.
- Relative lack of osteoporosis compared with rheumatoid arthritis.
- Sacroiliitis (Figs 47 & 48) and even fully established ankylosing spondylitis of identical or similar-type to that seen in idiopathic ankylosing spondylitis.

Laboratory features

Negative for rheumatoid factor. HLA Cw6 is associated with psoriasis, HLA DR7 with peripheral arthritis, HLA DR3 with erosive arthritis, and HLA B27 with sacroiliitis.

Management

- Integumentary features are managed as in the independent skin disorder.
- Rheumatic features—peripheral arthritis and/or spondylitis—are managed as in those conditions not associated with psoriasis, with some exceptions. Try to avoid corticosteroids and antimalarials; meticulous care should be taken to avoid postoperative sepsis.

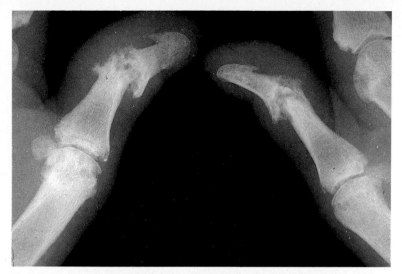

Fig. 46 Psoriatic arthritis. Typical changes; note phalangeal 'whittling' and 'cupping'.

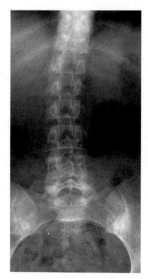

Fig. 47 Psoriatic arthritis. Early sacroiliitis/spondylitis.

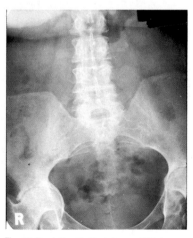

Fig. 48 Psoriatic arthritis. Late sacroiliitis/spondylitis.

6 / **Reiter's disease**

Definition The triad of arthritis, non-specific urethritis and conjunctivitis (named after H. Reiter, 1881–1969).

Prevalence Complicates about 1.7% of patients with non-specific urethritis and about 0.2% with dysentery. M:F = 20:1. Usual age of onset is about 20–40 yr.

Aetiology The condition is probably due to a combination of genetic and environmental factors. The latter being, at least in part, infections causing non-specific urethritis or, less commonly, cystitis, prostatitis (the genital type of Reiter's), dysentery or 'non-specific diarrhoea' (the intestinal type).

Clinical features **Acute stage**

- Urethritis (usual).
- Conjunctivitis (30%)—see Figure 49.
- Circinate balanitis (25%)—see Figure 50.
- Keratoderma blenorrhagica (15%)—see Figure 51.
- Erythema nodosum.
- Thrombophlebitis.
- Keratitis.
- Rheumatological manifestations (see p. 33).

Late stage

- Iritis (10%).
- Cardiac conduction defects and aortic incompetence (rare).
- Rheumatological manifestations (see p. 33).

Both the acute and later manifestations may be seen in other spondarthritides. For example, the skin lesions may be indistinguishable from pustular psoriasis, and the ocular features indistinguishable from those seen in ankylosing spondylitis or in the enteropathic arthropathies.

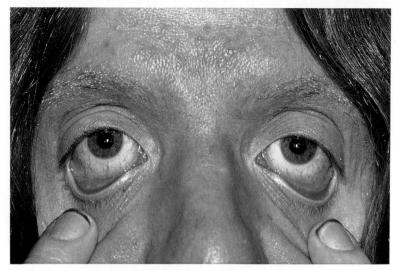

Fig. 49 Reiter's disease. Bilateral conjunctivitis.

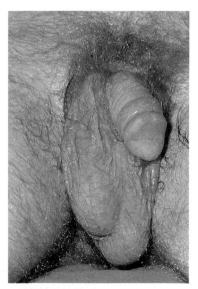

Fig. 50 Reiter's disease. Circinate balanitis.

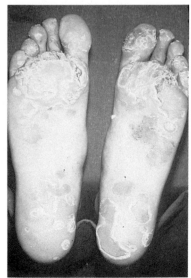

Fig. 51 Reiter's disease. Keratoderma blenorrhagica.

Clinical features
(contd)

Rheumatological manifestations
In addition to arthritis, patients may develop tenosynovitis, usually affecting the Achilles tendon (Fig. 52). In about the same frequency (20%), plantar fasciitis may occur.

Arthritis
Occurs up to about 4 weeks after infection. Knee (90%) and ankle (75%) are commonest patterns (Fig. 53). Feet are also often affected (40%). Shoulder, wrist, elbow, hip and spine are less often involved (30%). The arthritis is usually asymmetrical (75%) and polyarticular (90%), and may be migratory. The spinal involvement—sacroiliitis or fully developed ankylosing spondylitis—is in general of the type seen in other spondarthritides, with the exception shown in Figure 54.

Radiological
features

- Peripheral joints may be eroded or ankylosed, but often the arthritis is non-destructive.
- 'Fluffy' periosteal new bone formation—calcaneal spurs—and periosteal changes around the wrists, ankles or pelvis.
- Typical changes of ankylosing spondylitis in sacroiliac and intervertebral joints.
- 'Bridge lesions' (Fig. 54) not seen in other spondarthritides.

Laboratory
features

These include a much raised ESR and a negative rheumatoid factor. Patients with sacroiliitis are positive for HLA B27.

Management

- Treatment of arthritis and spondylitis along routine lines. (Phenylbutazone is particularly helpful.)
- Treatment of associated features and complications. It is worth trying oxytetracycline for genital infection, but the response may be disappointing.

There may be concomitant infection with gonococcus (50%).

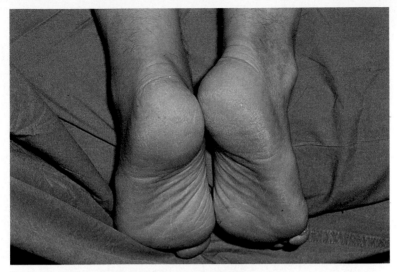

Fig. 52 Reiter's disease. Achilles tendinitis involving left ankle.

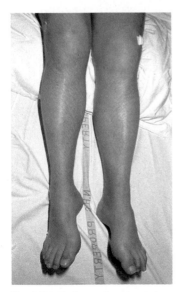

Fig. 53 Reiter's disease. Asymmetrical lowerlimb arthropathy.

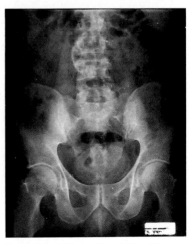

Fig. 54 Reiter's disease. Spondylitis with 'bridge lesion' and early sacroiliitis.

7 / Enteropathic arthropathies

Definition Arthropathy associated with ulcerative colitis, Crohn's disease or Whipple's disease.

Ulcerative colitis About 12% of patients with ulcerative colitis (typical barium features are shown in Fig. 55) develop an arthropathy. This is usually a monarticular acute synovitis, but occasionally polyarticular, most often affecting the knees, closely followed by the ankles. Shoulders, elbows, wrists and small joints of hands and feet are affected less often. The arthritis is non-erosive. It develops either at the onset of colitis or during its course. 'Parallelism' exists between exacerbations of colitis and joint disease. About 30% have sacroiliitis (Fig. 55), some of whom have typical ankylosing spondylitis. Associated features include erythema nodosum, thrombophlebitis, uveitis and digital clubbing.

Crohn's disease The typical barium features of Crohn's disease (named after B. B. Crohn, born 1884) are shown in Figure 56. The features of the arthropathy and the associated features are similar to those described for ulcerative colitis and affect mainly lower limb joints (Fig. 57). (The figure also shows the severe emaciation that may occur from malabsorption.) Sacroiliitis and spondylitis occur with roughly the same frequency as in colitis, and the features are the same (Fig. 58).

Whipple's disease Named after G. H. Whipple (1878–1976) and sometimes termed intestinal lipodystrophy, this is a much rarer disease than ulcerative colitis or Crohn's disease. It may be associated with peripheral and spinal arthritis of the type described above.

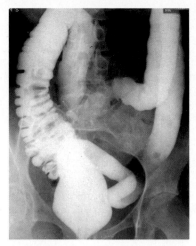

Fig. 55 Ulcerative colitis. Barium enema showing 'featureless' colon. Note also fused left sacroiliac joint.

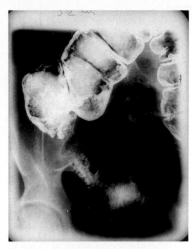

Fig. 56 Crohn's disease. Barium follow-through showing the 'string' sign of terminal ileitis.

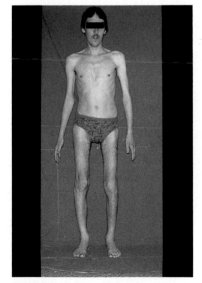

Fig. 57 Crohn's disease. Emaciation and synovitis affecting the left ankle.

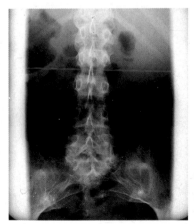

Fig. 58 Crohn's disease. Sacroiliitis and thoracolumbar syndesmophytes.

8 / Behçet's syndrome

Definition A disorder also known as Behçet's disease (after H. Behçet, 1889–1948), the triple symptom complex, or the cutaneo-muco-uveal syndrome. It is characterized by the simultaneous or successive occurrence of genital ulceration, oral ulceration, and uveitis or iridocyclitis.

Prevalence Rare. The condition is probably more common on Mediterranean littoral and in Japan. M:F = 2:1. Peak onset is in the third decade.

Aetiology Not known. Some believe it is related to the spondarthritides, some to the vasculitides. Familial in 30%.

Clinical features **Rheumatic manifestations**
Inflammatory lower limb arthropathy is seen, affecting the knees most often (75%) and ankles. It is monarticular in 10%, and may be migratory.

Associated features
These include aphthous ulcers (100%); genital ulcers (75%); uveitis (75%) (Fig. 59); skin lesions—erythema nodosum (Fig. 60), (skin particularly scrotal) ulceration (Fig. 61), sepsis (useful test based on puncture of skin which produces a pustule); thrombophlebitis or thrombosis (25%); CNS manifestations (10%); gastrointestinal (GI) manifestations (50%) and pulmonary lesions.

Radiological features Peripheral joints are normal. There is disagreement regarding sacroiliitis.

Laboratory features Raised ESR; leucocytosis; hyperglobulinaemia; rheumatoid factor negative and increased HLA B5. Biopsy may show vasculitis.

Management ● Symptomatic.
● Try corticosteroids and/or immunosuppressives for severe ocular or CNS disease.
● Avoid needle puncture if possible.

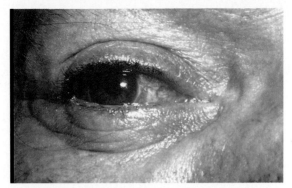

Fig. 59 Behçet's syndrome. Acute anterior uveitis.

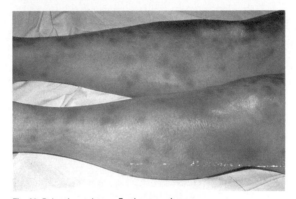

Fig. 60 Behçet's syndrome. Erythema nodosum.

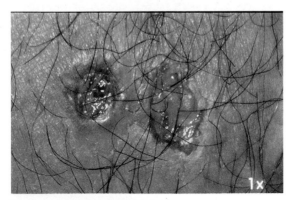

Fig. 61 Behçet's syndrome. Scrotal ulcers.

9 / Systemic lupus erythematosus (SLE)

Definition A disorder associated with multisystem involvement and characterized by the presence of antinuclear factor and other autoantibodies.

Prevalence Relatively common (probably about 0.5 per 1 000). The condition is more common in women (F:M = 9:1) and American negroes. Peak age of onset: 20–40 yr.

Aetiology As with many other systemic connective tissue diseases to be described the aetiology is unknown. Immunological factors are prominent, and there is strong evidence that immune complexes are filtered out of the circulation and are deposited in the basement membrane of the kidney and at other sites affected by the disease.

Clinical features **Joint involvement**
This occurs in over 90% cases and varies in presentation from flitting arthralgia to arthropathy similar to rheumatoid arthritis (Fig. 62). Progressive erosive changes are rare. Aseptic necrosis may occur.

Skin involvement
Sometimes there is a cutaneous vasculitis with overlap features of the type seen in systemic sclerosis or dermatomyositis. In the fingers a typical combination is telangiectasia of the base of the nail (Fig. 63) with digital erythema. The erythema is often more generalized (Fig. 64), affecting the hands, face and other parts. The most characteristic appearance is the 'butterfly' distribution of erythema on the cheeks and across the bridge of the nose (Fig. 64).

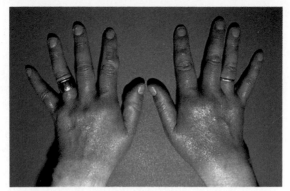

Fig. 62 SLE. Rheumatoid-pattern arthropathy.

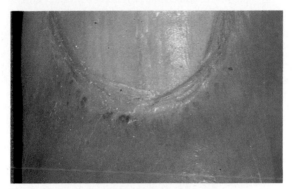

Fig. 63 SLE. Prominent nailfold capillaries.

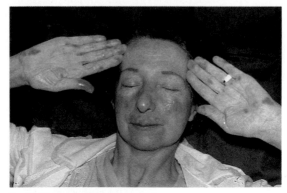

Fig. 64 SLE. Typical erythematous rash.

Clinical features
(contd)

Figure 65 shows this rash in another patient in further detail. Alopecia (Fig. 66), photosensitivity, Raynaud's phenomenon and subcutaneous nodules may also be seen.

Involvement of other systems
This includes renal disease (65%) with proteinuria, nephrotic syndrome and renal failure; lymphadenopathy (45%); hepatomegaly (40%); splenomegaly (25%); pleurisy with or without effusion (40%); pericarditis with or without tamponade (25%) (Fig. 67) and cardiac murmurs. Retinal cytoid bodies (10%) (Fig. 68), CNS manifestations (fits, psychoses, stroke, chorea) and peripheral neuropathy are also seen.

Radiological features

Joints are usually normal. X-ray manifestations of associated features can be seen.

Laboratory features

These include tests to identify circulating auto-antibodies directed against nuclear antigens (LE cell test; fluorescent antinuclear antibody, ANA; DNA-antibody tests—by immunochemical or immunofluorescent means). *Other tests* include those for other auto-antibodies and serum complement level. ESR is raised. Immunoglobulins are raised. Leucopenia is present. Skin biopsy can be examined by fluorescent techniques to detect immunoglobulin and complement deposition at dermo-epidermal junction.

Management

Corticosteroids are the mainstay of treatment. Antimalarials or an immunosuppressive agent (e.g. azathioprine) may be necessary. Treatment of associated disorders is important.

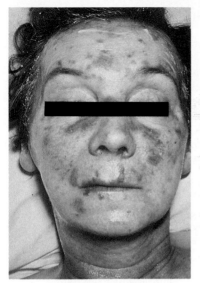

Fig. 65 SLE. Typical 'butterfly' rash.

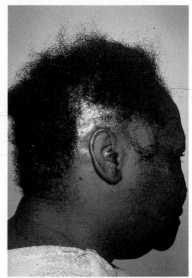

Fig. 66 SLE. Alopecia.

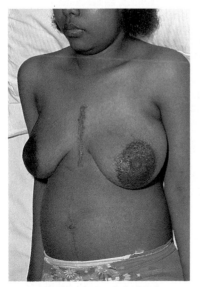

Fig. 67 SLE. Scar from surgical relief of pericardial tamponade.

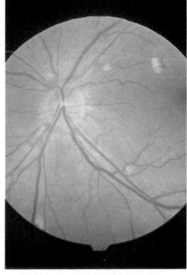

Fig. 68 SLE. 'Cytoid bodies' (exudates).

10 / **Progressive systemic sclerosis (scleroderma)**

Definition   A multisystem disorder characterized mainly by inflammation of subcutaneous connective tissue, followed by progressive fibrosis leading to atrophy of skin, subcutaneous fat and associated tissues, and arteritis of skin vessels.

Prevalence   Rare (about 9 per 100 000 females; 5 per 100 000 males). Peak age of onset: 30–50 yr.

Aetiology   Unknown, but there is strong clinical and serological overlap with other connective tissue disorders.

Clinical features   A typical clinical progression is for a young to middle-aged women to develop Raynaud's syndrome, followed by hardening of the skin of the fingers and mild arthritis of the knuckle joints. These features may be followed by involvement of internal organs such as the oesophagus. Further clinical details can be summarised thus:

- *Arthritis:* mild synovitis of finger joints resembling early rheumatoid arthritis. Combined with oedema of the skin and flexor tenosynovitis, the fingers may assume a sausage shape.
- *Skin changes:* vary from mild thickening and induration of the finger tips (acrosclerosis, sclerodactyly) to more widespread involvement affecting arms, upper trunk and face. Telangiectasia commonly accompanies the skin changes (Figs 69, 70 & 71). In addition to telangiectasia, the facies becomes characteristic, with a generalized 'pinched' look, microstomia and fissures radiating from the mouth (Fig. 72).

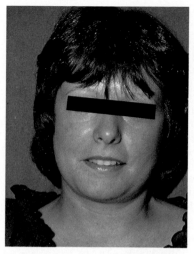

Fig. 69 Scleroderma. Facies in early disease. A few telangiectases on cheeks and neck.

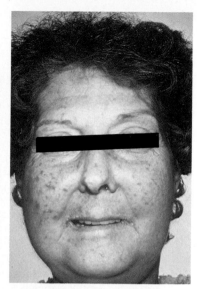

Fig. 70 Scleroderma. Prominent telangiectasia. 'Steroid facies'.

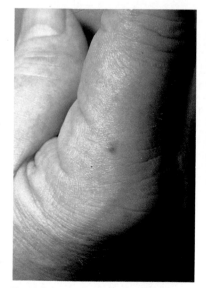

Fig. 71 Scleroderma. Detail of telangiectatic 'spider'.

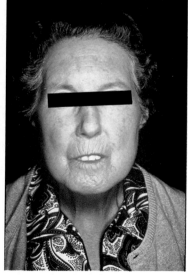

Fig. 72 Scleroderma. Facies in advanced disease. Note circumoral puckering and 'pinched' appearance.

Clinical features
(contd)

The appearance of the hands also becomes characteristic due to hardening and thickening of the skin, which produces a taut marble-like appearance with loss of skin creases and clawing (Fig. 73). Other skin features include pigmentation and ulceration of finger tips, knuckles or lower legs. Skin ulceration is associated with subcutaneous calcification in which subcuticular calcific nodules may discharge throught the skin (Fig. 74).

- *Visceral changes:* include Raynaud's phenomenon (common); dysphagia (65%), malabsorption or hepatic fibrosis; renal endarteritis with renal failure (20%); Sjögren's syndrome (6%); and rarely fibrosing alveolitis, myocardial fibrosis, pericarditis and other cardiac defects.

Radiological
features

- Resorption of distal phalanges (Fig. 75).
- Subcutaneous calcification (Fig. 75).
- Evidence of joint disease—joint space narrowing, periarticular osteoporosis, but no erosions.
  Barium swallow will show oesophageal changes.

Laboratory
features

These include a modest rise in ESR and in serum globulins, and a positive rheumatoid factor in 30%. Most patients have positive fluorescent antinuclear antibody tests.

Management

No really effective treatment is available. Advice is important for patients with Raynaud's phenomenon. Analgesic/anti-inflammatory drugs are used for synovitis. Systemic complications will require their own management.

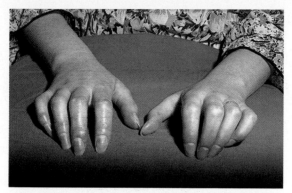

Fig. 73 Scleroderma. Sclerodactyly. Note 'creasless', clawed and slightly swollen fingers.

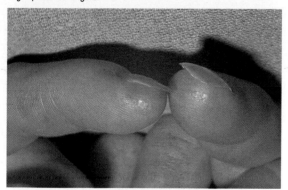

Fig. 74 Scleroderma. Calcinosis cutis.

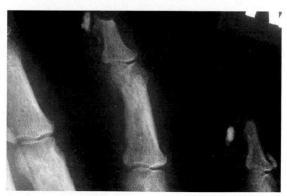

Fig. 75 Scleroderma. Acro-osteolysis with calcific deposits.

11 / Polyarteritis nodosa

Definition   A disorder in which widespread focal panarteritis with fibrinoid necrosis of the vessel wall produces multisystem disease—particularly affecting the kidneys, heart and nerves.

Prevalence   Rare. The exact prevalence is not known but it is less than 1:3 500. M:F = 4:1. The disorder is rare under age 20 and over age 65.

Aetiology   Unknown, but there is evidence for an immunological disturbance, with deposition of immune complexes in vessel walls.

Clinical features   A serious disease with widespread clinical manifestations.
- *'Rheumatological':* generalized muscle/joint pains (70%); arthritis (25%). This may be acute (resembling rheumatic fever) or chronic (resembling RA). Hypertrophic osteoarthropathy may also occur.
- *Other features:* systemic disturbance (fever, weight loss, malaise); renal disease (90%); peripheral neuropathy (50%); cardiovascular disease, including hypertension (50%), heart failure, acute pericarditis (30%) and painless myocardial infarction (common); lung involvement (30%); skin lesions (25%), including purpura, bruising, livedo reticularis (Fig. 76), dermal infarction (Fig. 77) or more extensive gangrene (Fig. 78); GI involvement and CNS disease.

Radiological features   In chronic forms, joint changes are as in RA. Selective renal angiography may show arterial aneurysms.

Laboratory features   These include raised ESR, neutrophil leucocytosis, absolute eosinophilia (especially with lung involvement), mild anaemia and hypergammaglobulinaemia. Rheumatoid factor is positive in 30%. Biopsy of clinically involved tissues is positive in about 40%. Characteristic features (Fig. 79) include arterial fibrinoid necrosis and inflammatory cells.

Management   Corticosteroids and immunosuppressive drugs (e.g. azathioprine), but response may be poor.

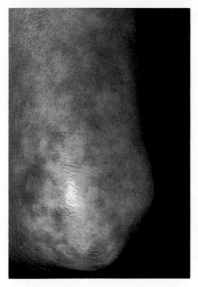

Fig. 76 Polyarteritis nodosa. Livedo reticularis on elbow region.

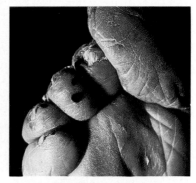

Fig. 77 Polyarteritis nodosa. Dermal infarcts on toes.

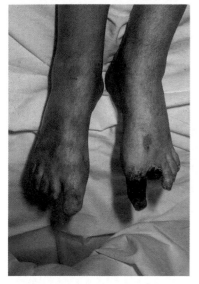

Fig. 78 Polyarteritis nodosa. Gangrene of toes.

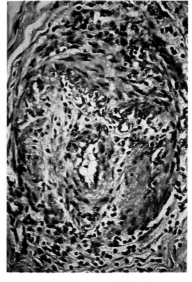

Fig. 79 Polyarteritis nodosa. Biopsy showing widespread fibrinoid necrosis and inflammatory cells.

12 / **Polymyositis and dermatomyositis**

Definition	*Polymyositis* refers to acquired inflammatory disorders of voluntary muscles, proximal weakness being the main feature. When this is associated with skin involvement, the term *dermatomyositis* is used.
Prevalence	Rare. F:M = 3:1.
Aetiology	An immunological disturbance. The relationship with virus infection and triggering by malignant disease is still not clear.

Clinical features

The clinical presentation may be divided into childhood and adult dermatomyositis. The latter generally develops in the mid-adult years and may be further divided into:

- Pure polymyositis, with voluntary muscle weakness affecting mainly proximal limb and girdle muscles.
- Polymyositis with features of other connective tissue diseases.
- Other connective tissue disorders with incidental polymyositis.
- Mixed connective tissue disease—'overlap syndromes', e.g. polymyositis + systemic lupus erythematosus + systemic sclerosis.
- Adult dermatomyositis (Figs 80–82).

Radiological features

The joints are normal. Calcification of skin and proximal limb muscles is seen.

Laboratory features

These include raised ESR (50%) and raised muscle enzymes (75%)—creatine kinase and aldolase most specific for diagnosis and useful for monitoring treatment. Typical muscle biopsy is seen in 75%. EMG is usually abnormal but not specific. Rheumatoid factor is positive in 50%, and ANF positive in 30%.

Management

- Corticosteroids—if no response one of the remission-inducing agents (e.g. gold, penicillamine, antimalarials).
- Physiotherapy to improve muscle function.

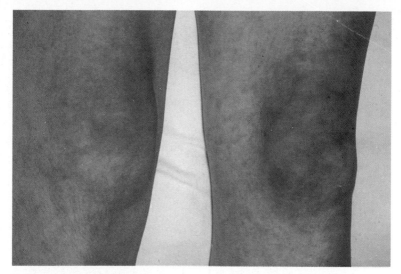

Fig. 80 Dermatomyositis. Erythema on knees.

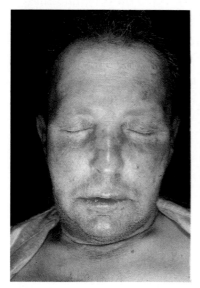

Fig. 81 Dermatomyositis. Periorbital heliotrope rash.

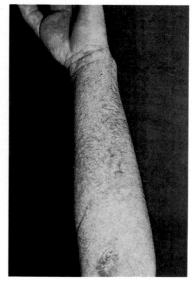

Fig. 82 Dermatomyositis. Scaly rash on elbow and forearm.

13 / Osteoarthrosis

Definition	Osteoarthrosis (syn. osteoarthritis, OA) is a degenerative disease of synovial joints, commonly associated with minor inflammatory features due to a primary cartilage disorder.
Prevalence	Very common, affecting about 20% of the population. F:M = 2:1. Peak age of onset: 50 yr. About 50% of the population have radiological changes of OA but only half of these have symptoms.
Aetiology	Not known. Genetic factors are probably important in some types. The cartilage disturbance leads to:

- roughening ('fibrillation') and wearing (thinning) of the cartilage surface (leading to exposure of underlying bone)
- impairment of the cushioning 'shock-absorber' function (leading to damage of underlying bone).

Clinical features   **Joints affected:** knees (75%) and hands (60%)—commonest. In the hands, involvement of the DIP joints and carpometacarpal joints gives rise to typical features (Fig. 83). The DIP joint swellings—Heberden's nodes (after W. Heberden, 1710–1801) are pathognomic and are shown in more detail in Figure 84. Swellings involving PIP joint are called Bouchard's nodes. The feet are involved in 40%; usually the 1st MTP joint. Hips (25%), ankles (20%), shoulders (15%), and lumbar (30%) and cervical spine (20%) are also affected. When involvement affects a less usual site, in the absence of OA elsewhere, secondary OA should be considered as in Figure 85.

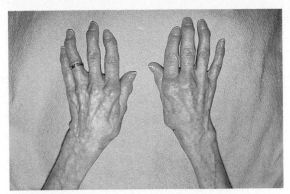

Fig. 83 OA. DIP joint deformities and hand 'squaring' (carpometacarpal arthritis of thumbs).

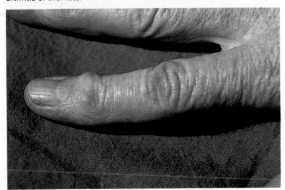

Fig. 84 OA. Heberden's nodes.

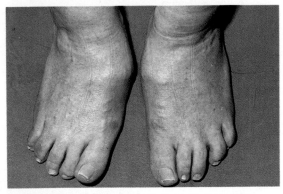

Fig. 85 OA. Bony prominence over tarsal joints due to secondary osteoarthrosis.

Clinical features
(contd)

Symptoms: pain worse towards evening and aggravated by particular activities. Characteristically, there is immobility or inactivity stiffness ('gelling'), but morning stiffness may be present.

Signs: bony swelling, soft swelling if effusion present, crepitus, painful limitation of movement and deformity. Baker's cysts or other synovial cysts (e.g. suprapatellar) may occur.

Course: slowly progressive with exacerbations and remissions. Greatest problems arise from involvement of weight-bearing joints. No systemic features.

Radiological features

- Loss of joint space.
- Sclerosis of adjacent bone.
- Osteophytes.
- Subarticular cysts.

These changes can be seen in various joints in the accompanying figures—thumbs (Fig. 86), big toe (Fig. 87), knee (Fig. 88) and hip (Fig. 89). Sometimes articular calcification is an associated feature. Occasionally erosions or ankylosis are present ('erosive OA'), but this may be a different disease.

Laboratory features

No diagnostic tests.

Management

As for chronic arthritis, generally:

- Analgesic or analgesic/anti-inflammatory drugs.
- Physiotherapy.
- Aids and appliances.
- Surgery.

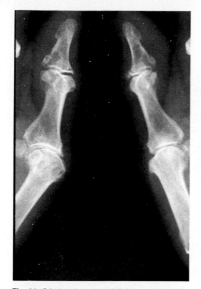

Fig. 86 OA. Involvement of IP joints of thumb.

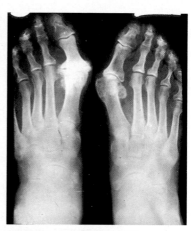

Fig. 87 OA. Involvement of 1st MTP joints, left more than right.

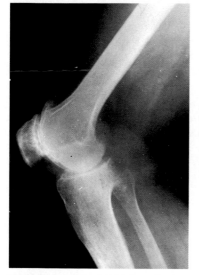

Fig. 88 OA. Involvement of tibiofemoral and patellofemoral joints.

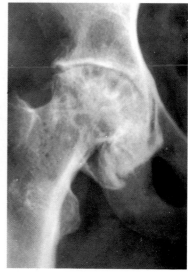

Fig. 89 OA. Hip joint involvement (osteophytes, cysts, sclerosis, and joint-space narrowing).

14 / Spondylosis

Definition	Essentially a radiological concept, it refers to all degenerative changes in the spine. Some restrict the term to degenerative changes involving intervertebral as opposed to facetal (synovial) joints (the latter being classed under 'osteoarthrosis').
Prevalence	Very common (see p. 57).
Aetiology	Often follows disc prolapse but aetiology not clear (see p. 57).
Clinical features	Chronic pain, slight stiffness and root symptoms (see p. 57). In the neck, vertebral artery compression and spinal canal stenosis may occur. Spinal stenosis may also occur in the lumbar region and cause 'neurogenic claudication' due to ischaemia of the cauda equina.
Radiological features	Features identical with osteoarthrosis, notably osteophytes and joint space narrowing. The osteophytes are beak-like (Figs 90–93), may be fused and, when marked, give the spine a gnarled appearance. They must be distinguished from the bony outgrowths of ankylosing spondylitis (these are slimmer and more vertical) and those of ankylosing hyperostosis (these are more exuberant and can involve the entire height of vertebral bodies and not just their marginal lips).
Laboratory features	Unhelpful.
Management	See page 57 for general principles. Surgery may be required for relief of cord compression or osteophyte encroachment on a nerve root.

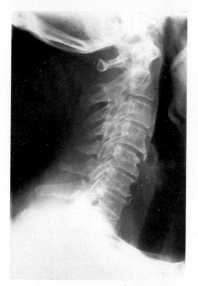

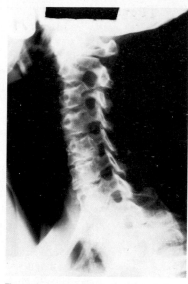

Fig. 90 Spondylosis. Cervical osteophytes and disc space narrowing (Lateral view.)

Fig. 91 Spondylosis. Narrowing of cervical intervertebral foramina. (Oblique view.)

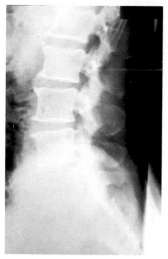

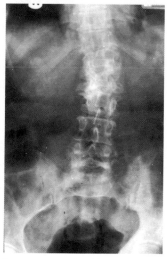

Fig. 92 Spondylosis. Lumbar osteophytes. (Lateral view.)

Fig. 93 Spondylosis. Massive lumbar osteophytes with disc space loss and scoliosis. (AP view.)

15 / Disc lesions

Definition This term covers a wide range of lesions from acute disc protrusion in younger patients, to shrinkage of multiple discs and secondary bony overgrowth in older patients.

Prevalence Very common, increases with age. After age 60 it is rare to find a completely normal spine on X-ray.

Aetiology In acute cases the annulus fibrosus tears, allowing the nucleus pulposus to herniate. Later, the water content of the disc decreases and it shrinks. Genetic and occupational factors are probably involved.

Clinical features Acute disc protrusion causes local pain, root symptoms and sometimes signs, limited spinal bending and scoliosis (Fig. 94). Disc shrinkage and bony overgrowth may also cause local pain and root problems. The commonest spinal segments affected are the lower cervical and lower lumbar regions. The former gives rise to neck pain and 'brachialgia', and the latter to 'lumbago' and 'sciatica'. Rarely, central (as opposed to posterolateral) protrusion occurs, causing cord compression in the cervical region and cauda equina entrapment in the lumbar region.

Radiological features
- *Plain X-ray:* reduced disc space with or without secondary bony overgrowth. Vertical herniations appear as Schmorl's nodes.
- *Myelography:* indentation of Myodil column (Fig. 95).
- *Discography:* degenerate disc (normal has central bilobed nucleus).

Laboratory features Unhelpful.

Management Cervical and lumbar disc problems are managed with pain relief; rest in bed with or without collar or corset, and with or without traction (Fig. 96) in acute phase; preventative advice; and mobilization exercises in post-acute phase. Chymopapain injection of lumbar discs is still controversial; surgery (e.g. lumbar laminectomy) (Fig. 97) is indicated only in selected cases.

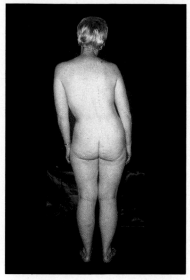

Fig. 94 Acute lumbar disc lesion. Scoliosis.

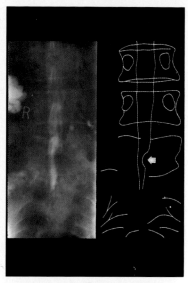

Fig. 95 Acute lumbar disc lesion. Myelogram showing indentation of Myodil column.

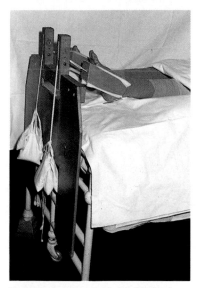

Fig. 96 Acute lumbar disc lesion. Details of leg traction apparatus.

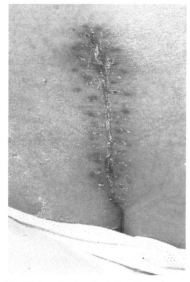

Fig. 97 Acute lumbar disc lesion. Site and extent of healing laminectomy scar.

16 / Gout

Definition and aetiology   A disease with a marked familial tendency, occurring mainly in adult men. It is characterized by episodes of acute arthritis, and later also by chronic arthritis and damage to soft tissues and kidney. It is caused essentially by an excess of urate in the blood (hyperuricaemia) and tissues.

Prevalence   Affects 3–4 per 1 000 (about the same frequency as ankylosing spondylitis). It is more prevalent in upper social classes, Polynesian races and alcohol drinkers. It affects men after puberty and women after the menopause.

Clinical features   Acute arthritis affects the big toe (MTR joint) in 75% of attacks (Fig. 98). Occasionally, ankle, other toes, knee or finger (Fig. 99) are affected. Sometimes the disease affects more than one joint (Fig. 100), but it is monarticular in 90%. The joint is exquisitely painful, red, hot, swollen and very tender. Skin peeling occurs after acute attack, and fever is common. Untreated acute attacks last for a few days or weeks, and recur at irregular intervals, sometimes many years apart. Between attacks joints are normal. Later the arthritis becomes chronic and is associated with deformity and tophaceous deposits (Fig. 101).

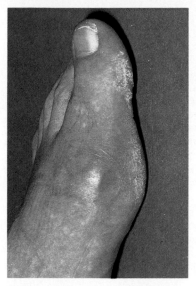

Fig. 98 Gout. Acute arthritis: dusky, shiny erythema overlying swollen 1st MTP joint.

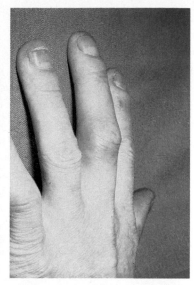

Fig. 99 Gout. Acute arthritis: erythema and swelling of 3rd PIP joint.

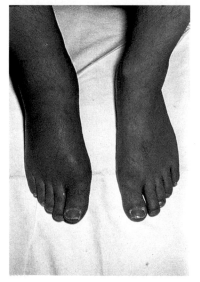

Fig. 100 Gout. Acute arthritis: multiple joint involvement of left foot and ankle.

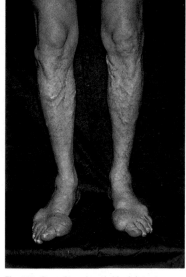

Fig. 101 Gout. Chronic arthritis: joint deformities associated with massive tophi.

Clinical features (contd) Tophi are found in 20% of patients, characteristically in the helix of the pinna (Fig. 102). Other sites include the olecranon and prepatellar bursae, and tendons. Tophi may ulcerate and exude chalky urate salts (Fig. 103). The surrounding inflammation and discharging material may suggest an infected joint, as in the patient shown in Figure 103.

Associated clinical conditions: obesity (50%); hypertension (50%), vascular disease, and renal failure; renal uric acid stones.

Variants: secondary gout (e.g. myeloproliferative disorders during treatment of malignant disease); renal failure (e.g. lead poisoning—saturnine gout, hyperparathyroidism, hypothyroidism); Lesch–Nyhan syndrome (inherited disorder of urate metabolism); glycogen storage disease.

Radiological features 'Punched-out' radiolucent areas around joints in which there are tophaceous deposits (Fig. 104).

Laboratory features
- Synovial fluid and tophi contain needle-shaped crystals (Fig. 105). These are strongly negatively birefringent under polarized light.
- Serum uric acid usually greater than 0.36 mmol/l (6 mg%). It is wise to do a series of values.
- Raised ESR and leucocytosis in acute phase.

Management *Acute attacks:* full dosage of indomethacin or other non-steroidal anti-inflammatory drug (e.g. naproxen). Long-term therapy with urate-lowering drugs (uricosurics or allopurinol) may be needed.

Indications: frequent attacks, serum uric acid > 0.54 mmol/l (9 mg%), tophi and renal stones.

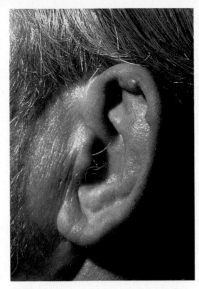

Fig. 102 Gout. Tophi in classical site on helix of ear.

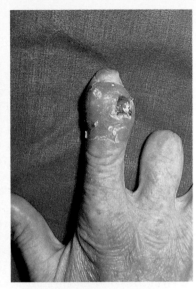

Fig. 103 Gout. Ulcerating tophus associated with chronic gouty arthritis of 2nd DIP joint.

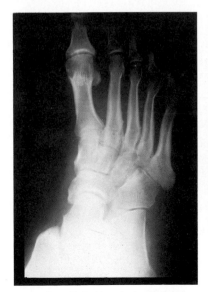

Fig. 104 Gout. Typical 'punched out' erosions of 1st MTP joint due to tophaceous deposits.

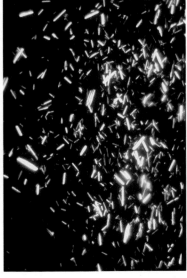

Fig. 105 Gout. Needle-shaped uric acid crystals.

17 / **Pseudogout**

Definition A condition otherwise known as pyrophosphate arthropathy, pseudogout is associated with deposition of crystals of calcium pyrophosphate dihydrate into joints. The term chondrocalcinosis (a typical feature of pseudogout) should be reserved for the radiological appearance of linear calcification of articular cartilage.

Prevalence M = F. Age of onset: 30+ yr, typically over 60 yr. Earlier onset in familial cases. In elderly patients, a 7–28% frequency of meniscal calcification has been reported.

Aetiology Less is known about the aetiology and pathogenesis of pseudogout than urate gout, but there are similarities between the two diseases in respect of familial tendency, provoking factors, and pattern of disease expression.

Clinical features Clinical patterns of arthritis are as follows: pseudogout; pseudorheumatoid arthritis; pseudo-osteoarthrosis; pseudo-osteoarthritis with superimposed acute attacks; asymptomatic pyrophosphate deposits; pseudo-neurotrophic joints.

  The knee is the commonest joint to be affected, and the acute features resemble gout. The chronic features resemble OA.

Radiological features Linear calcification of cartilage (Figs 106 & 107) and degenerative changes indistinguishable from OA.

Laboratory features ***Synovial fluid:*** brick-shaped crystals (Fig. 108) which are weakly positively birefringent under polarized light.
Blood: raised ESR and leucocytosis in acute attacks.

Management ***Acute stage:*** aspiration and injection with steroid; analgesic/anti-inflammatory drugs; rest.
Chronic stage: as for osteoarthrosis.

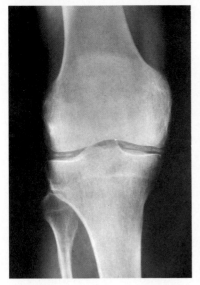

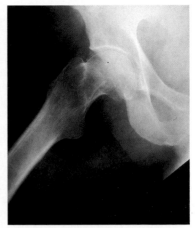

Fig. 106 Pseudogout. Chondrocalcinosis of knee joint articular cartilage.

Fig. 107 Pseudogout. Chondrocalcinosis of hip joint articular cartilage.

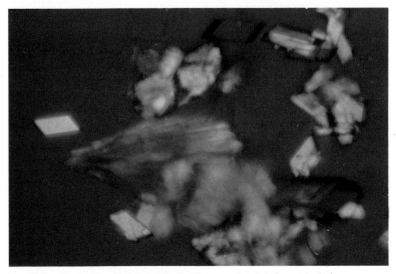

Fig. 108 Pseudogout. Rhomboidal crystals of calcium pyrophosphate (grown *in vitro*).

18 / Septic (suppurative) arthritis

Definition   Infection of a joint with pyogenic (pus-forming) bacteria.

Prevalence   M:F = 2:1 Seen particularly in children and the elderly.

Aetiology   The commonest causative organism is *Staphylococcus aureus* (50%). *Streptococcus pyogenes, Strep. faecalis, Strep. viridans, E. coli, Haemophilus influenzae, Proteus, Pseudomonas aeruginosa, Klebsiella, Aerobacter, Vibrio fetus* and *Serratia* may cause the same clinical picture. It is rarely a complication of infection elsewhere. There is usually (70%) a predisposing factor (e.g. RA, diabetes mellitus, joint paracentesis or surgery, steroid therapy or debilitating disease).

Clinical features   The knee is most commonly affected (50%), though sometimes other joints are affected (see Fig. 109). Monarticular in 90%. The pain is severe, and the joint is very tender, warm, red and swollen. Fever is usual.

Radiological features   Osteoporosis appears after about 2 weeks. Thereafter, destructive changes may progress rapidly (Fig. 110). Leucocytosis is seen in 90%.

Laboratory features   Macroscopically, joint aspiration (or drainage via a scalpel incision) reveals thick yellow-green pus (Fig. 111). Synovial fluid WBC > $30\,000 \times 10^9$/dl, 90% neutrophils. Gram stain is positive in 50%, and culture positive in 85%. If negative, repeat for anaerobic culture.

Management
- Appropriate antibiotic (oral or i.m.).
- Rest.
- Daily aspiration.
- Physiotherapy to restore joint function.

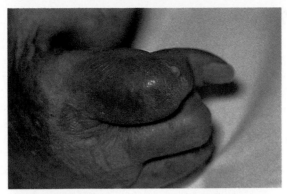

Fig. 109 Septic arthritis. Pus exuding from infected PIP joint.

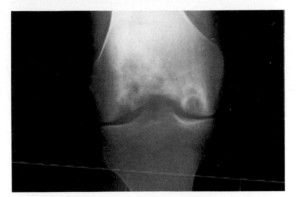

Fig. 110 Septic arthritis. Large rapidly developing erosions of femoral condyles.

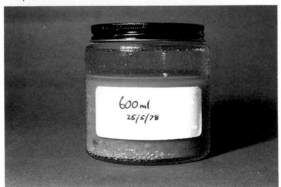

Fig. 111 Septic arthritis. Pus drained from infected knee joint and related calf cyst.

19 / Gonococcal arthritis

Definition and aetiology	Arthritis due to infection of joints with *Neisseria gonorrhoeae*.
Prevalence	Becoming more common. F:M = 4:1. The infection is seen at any age, but particularly in young adults. Male patients are often homosexual. Of those with gonococcal urethritis, 0.2% develop arthritis.
Clinical features	Useful points in favour of gonococcal polyarthritis, as opposed to Reiter's disease, are:

- Patient often female.
- Upper, as well as lower, limb joints involved.
- Often involvement of 'unusual' joints (e.g. superior tibiofibular joint).
- Characteristic pustular skin lesions.
- Response to antibiotics.

In view of importance of rash in diagnosis, several Figures showing this are included (Figs 112–115). The rash occurs in 70% of patients with arthritis and may be maculopapular, haemorrhagic, vesicular or pustular (as here), particularly in the limbs.

Radiological features	Normal in acute stage. Erosive changes may occur later.
Laboratory features	Synovial fluid culture is positive in 50%. The organism may also be recovered from blood, the genital tract, anus or pharynx.
Management	

- Penicillin. If hypersensitive or resistant, try tetracycline.
- Counselling and examination of contacts.

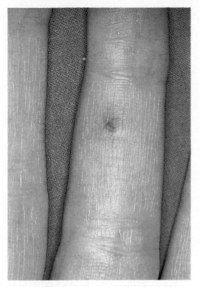

Fig. 112 Gonococcal arthritis. Small pustule on finger.

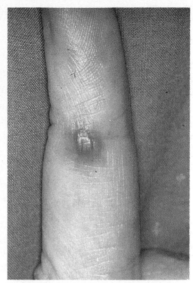

Fig. 113 Gonococcal arthritis. Larger pustule on finger—note erythematous base.

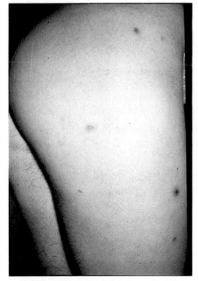

Fig. 114 Gonococcal arthritis. Crop of healing pustules on buttocks and thighs.

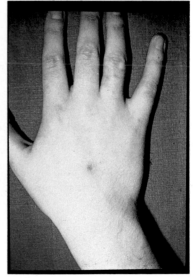

Fig. 115 Gonococcal arthritis. Isolated pustule on dorsum of hand.

20 / **Tuberculous arthritis**

Definition   Infection of joint or spine with *Mycobacterium tuberculosis.*

Prevalence   Now rare in UK. M > F. The infection is seen at any age, though it is commoner in children and elderly, particularly if debilitated or malnourished.

Aetiology   Joint involvement is usually secondary to involvement of bone. Rarely, direct involvement of synovium occurs.

Clinical features   Joints affected include the spine, particularly dorsal region (40%), and the hip (25%). It may also affect the knee (15%), ankle or foot (5%), and the sacroiliac joint (5%).

   The onset is insidious. Pain is minimal at first and often worse at the end of day. If untreated, the infection progresses rapidly to deformity and joint destruction. Discharging sinuses may develop.

Radiological features   Typical radiological changes associated with tuberculous peripheral arthritis are (Figs 116–119):

- Early: normal or osteoporosis.
- Later: diminished joint space.
- Erosions and rarely subarticular cysts with sclerotic margins.
- Smudgy irregular bone outline from destructive changes.
- Soft-tissue calcification in the healing phase.

Typically, the spine shows narrowing of intervertebral space due to disc destruction, and areas of osteoporosis and later destructive changes in adjacent vertebrae.

Laboratory   Bacterial confirmation is by direct examination, culture and guinea-pig inoculation using synovial fluid or biopsy material.

Management   Chemotherapy as for TB elsewhere, rest, traction or splintage, and surgical debridement.

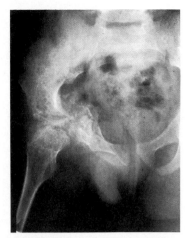

Fig. 116 Tuberculous arthritis. Involvement of hip with soft-tissue calcification.

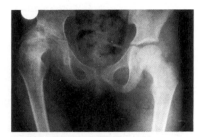

Fig. 117 Tuberculous arthritis. Long-standing right hip arthritis. Note hypoplasia.

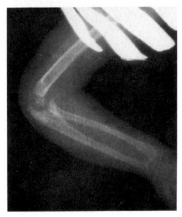

Fig. 118 Tuberculous arthritis. Involvement of elbow.

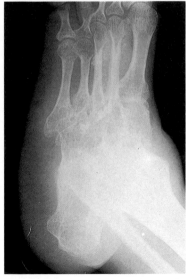

Fig. 119 Tuberculous arthritis. Involvement of tarsus and metatarsus. Note calcification.

21 / Hypertrophic osteoarthropathy/Digital clubbing

Hypertrophic arthropathy

The syndrome of digital clubbing, painful tender swelling of bones and joints (commonly the ankles and wrists) and radiological periostitis form the characteristic presentation. It may be due to:

- Benign or malignant, primary or secondary tumours of lung, pleura, heart, diaphragm, mediastinum, or upper GI tract.
- Pulmonary suppuration (bronchiectasis, lung abscess, empyema).
- Aortic aneurysm.
- GI disorder (ulcerative colitis, Crohn's disease, steatorrhoea, hepatic cirrhosis).
- Cyanotic congenital heart disease.
- An autosomal dominant disorder (rare).

Digital clubbing

Digital clubbing is an essential feature of hypertrophic osteoarthropathy (most commonly seen in middle-aged men with bronchial carcinoma), but it also occurs in:

- Pachydermoperiostosis (Touraine–Solente–Golé syndrome), a syndrome characterized by absence of other underlying disease, periostosis leading to enlargement of the extremities, thickening of the skin and scalp (pachydermia), and an arthropathy.
- Thyroid acropachy (see under hyperthyroidism, p. 83).

Clinical features are shown in Figure 120, with further detail shown in Figure 121. Apart from soft-tissue swelling of the terminal portions of the fingers (sometimes marked enough to justify the term 'drum-sticking'), the nails are curved longitudinally and horizontally, and the angle between nail plate and base of nail is obliterated.

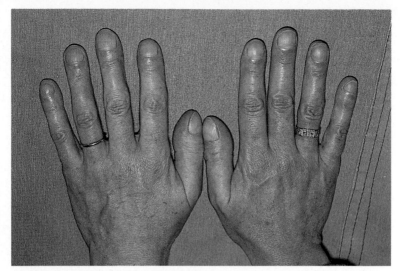

Fig. 120 Digital clubbing. Note all fingers affected.

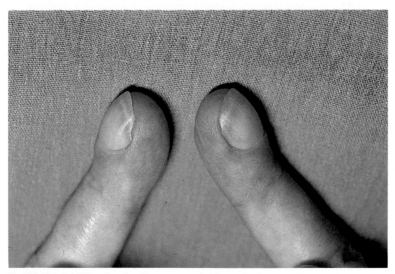

Fig. 121 Digital clubbing. Detail: nail curvature and obliterated nail plate/nail base angle.

22 / **Periostitis**

Definition   Periostitis (or periosteitis, but not periostosis) is a term to describe radiographic periosteal shadowing due to new bone deposition and calcification outside the bone cortex.

Clinical types   ● 'Onion-skin appearance'—periosteal new bone formed in layers with translucent tissue between them (e.g. secondary deposit from neuroblastoma).
● 'Sun-ray appearance'—subperiosteal calcification formed at right angles to the bone shaft (e.g. osteosarcoma).
● Narrow linear shadow running more or less parallel to the cortex (Figs 122–125). This is the most common appearance (e.g. periostitis of hypertrophic osteoarthropathy).

Aetiology   The causes of periosteal shadowing include: post-traumatic shadowing; non-traumatic haematoma; stress, fatigue or pseudofracture; inflammatory conditions (e.g. pyogenic, syphilitic, tuberculous or fungal infections of bone); benign neoplasms (e.g. osteoid osteoma); malignant neoplasms (e.g. Ewing's tumour); vascular disorders (varicose veins, arterial occlusion); hypertrophic osteoarthropathy (see p. 71); pachydermoperiostosis and melorheostosis.

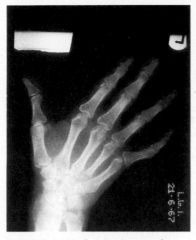

Fig. 122 Periostitis. Early involvement of phalanges and metacarpals. Radius and ulna also affected.

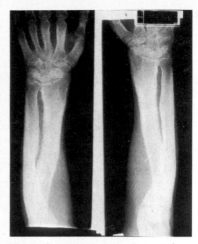

Fig. 123 Periostitis. Marked involvement of forearm bones, particularly radii.

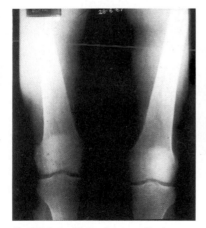

Fig. 124 Periostitis. Involvement of both femora.

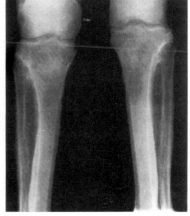

Fig. 125 Periostitis. Marked involvement of tibiae and fibulae. Femora also affected.

23 / **Malignancy**

Carcinoma arthritis

Definition
A rheumatic disorder clinically resembling RA, occurring in any type of malignant disease (particularly in carcinoma of the bronchus, prostate and breast), but not due to metastases in bone or joint.

Prevalence
M:F = 2:1. Peak age of onset: 50–65 yr.

Aetiology
Unknown. Mechanisms based on alterations of cellular immunity or circulating immune complexes have been suggested, but remain unproven.

Clinical features
Carcinoma arthritis may be the presenting feature of malignancy. In others, clinical features relating to a specific malignant condition will be present. Common examples of such features are shown in Figures 126–128.

- Onset typically about 1 yr before manifestation of malignancy.
- Joints affected: knees, ankles, MCP and MTP joints commonest; 20% monarticular; 50% asymmetrical. Joints may be warm, red, swollen and tender in acute stage.
- Course: variable, usually remits with control of malignancy.

Radiological features
Usually normal.

Laboratory features
Non-specific blood and synovial evidence of inflammation.

Management
- Control of associated malignant disease.
- Analgesic/anti-inflammatory drugs.

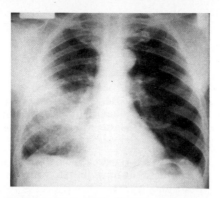

Fig. 126 Carcinoma arthritis. Underlying cause—bronchogenic carcinoma right lung.

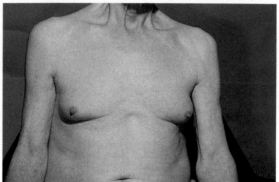

Fig. 127 Carcinoma arthritis. Underlying cause—prostatic carcinoma. Note gynaecomastia from stilboestrol therapy.

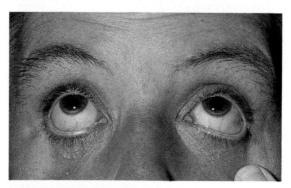

Fig. 128 Carcinoma arthritis. Underlying cause—pancreatic carcinoma presenting with jaundice.

Metastases

Definition   The term metastasis (Greek, a removing = *meta* + *stasis* = a placing) in reference to cancer denotes the appearance of neoplasms in parts remote from the primary tumour.

Clinical and radiological features   The clinico-radiological implications of skeletal metastases (most often from a bronchogenic carcinoma) in rheumatology are as follows:

- Pain from single or multiple metastases, often evident as osteolytic or osteosclerotic lesions on X-ray (Figs 129–132), may initially be ascribed to 'fibrositis' or other forms of soft-tissue rheumatism.
- Polyarthritis may result from metastatic invasion of joints. Usually asymmetrical.
- Symmetrical metastatic finger deposits may resemble RA. Picture may be additionally confusing if patients are seropositive for rheumatoid factor (20% with malignancy seropositive).
- Phalangeal metastases may simulate gout, osteomyelitis or tenosynovitis by direct synovial implantation or by involvement of juxta-articular bone.
- Involvement of the axial skeleton may mimic spondylosis with or without radiculopathy.

Management
- Treatment of rheumatic manifestations: symptomatically with analgesics or analgesic/anti-inflammatory drugs. Narcotic analgesics may be required.
- Treatment of the primary (if known) and secondary deposits if possible with chemotherapy and/or radiotherapy according to clinical circumstances.

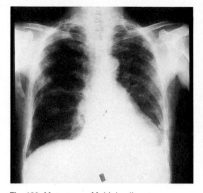

Fig. 129 Metastases. Multiple, discrete osteoblastic secondaries in ribs and scapulae.

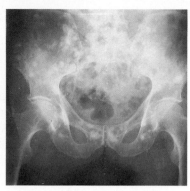

Fig. 130 Metastases. Multiple, discrete osteoblastic secondaries throughout pelvis.

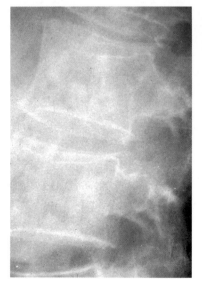

Fig. 131 Metastases. Patchy sclerosis due to secondaries in vertebrae.

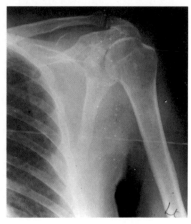

Fig. 132 Metastases. Isolated secondary in acromion—an unusual site.

Myelomatosis

Definition   Chronic, progressive, invariably fatal disorder due to malignant plasma cell proliferation characterized by the development of multiple bone tumours.

Prevalence   M:F = 2:1. Peak age of onset: 50–70 yr.

Aetiology   Unknown.

Clinical features   Bone pain occurs in 90%. Pain is localized to the joints in 15%. Three types of arthritis occur:
- Due to myeloma deposits in bone near joints.
- Associated with amyloidosis.
- Arthritis resembling carcinoma arthritis.

Additional rheumatic effects may arise from pathological fractures, nervous system involvement, chronic renal insufficiency and the effects of corticosteroids.

Radiological features   A classical X-ray finding is the 'pepper-pot skull' (Figs 133 & 134) due to osteolytic deposits. Similar deposits may occur near joints and in the pelvis. Osteoporosis is seen particularly in the spine and may, together with lytic lesions, cause vertebral collapse. Pathological fractures may also be revealed on X-ray.

Laboratory features   ESR is usually > 50 mm/h. Paraprotein on electrophoresis is seen in 75%; diminished immunoglobulin levels. Bence–Jones proteinuria is seen in 40%; hypercalcaemia in 50%. Bone-marrow aspiration reveals plasma-cell infiltration—confirmatory.

Management   Radiotherapy to painful areas; analgesic/anti-inflammatories and narcotics later if necessary.

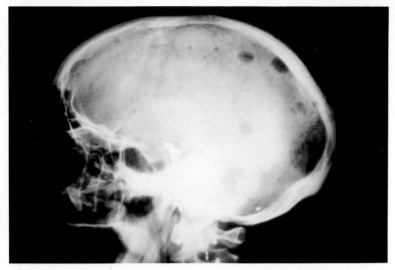

Fig. 133 Myelomatosis. 'Pepper-pot skull' showing multiple lytic deposits—lateral view.

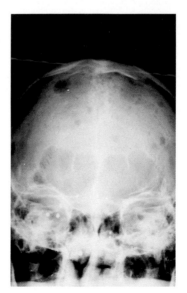

Fig. 134 Myelomatosis. 'Pepper-pot skull'—anteroposterior (AP) view.

24 / Endocrine disorders

Pituitary gigantism/acromegaly

Definition Pituitary adenomas causing chronic over-production of growth hormone cause gigantism before, and acromegaly after, epiphyseal closure.

Prevalence F:M = 3:2. Commonest age of acromegaly onset: 20–40 yr. 50% of acromegalics have arthropathy.

Aetiology Pituitary adenoma causes increased anabolism (mainly of collagen) and cellular proliferation (mainly fibroblastic).

Clinical features
- Before epiphyses close, gigantism due mainly to increased 'longitudinal' growth occurs. It may be associated with aches and pains, and postural changes, but there are no clear-cut rheumatic syndromes.
- After epiphyseal closure, longitudinal growth no longer being possible, 'horizontal' growth occurs, seen as gradual enlargement of the bones and soft tissues of the head (Figs 135 & 136), hands (Fig. 137) and feet. Main rheumatic features of acromegaly are: low backache; limb arthropathy (often knees); entrapment neuropathies (usually carpal tunnel syndrome); neuromuscular symptoms and Raynaud's phenomenon.

Radiological features These include tufting of distal phalanges; increased joint space; exostoses–phalangeal 'lips' and 'hooks' and spinal osteophytes; calcification of joint capsule and cartilage; thickened, widely-spaced trabeculae and enlarged pituitary fossa.

Laboratory features Insulin and glucose-tolerance tests, and growth hormone level are confirmatory.

Management
- Treatment of adenoma (hypophysectomy), but this has no effect on arthropathy.
- Analgesics.
- Carpal tunnel decompression.

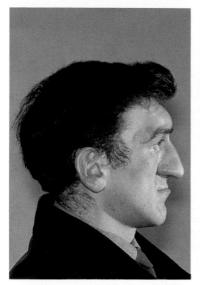

Fig. 135 Acromegaly. Typical facies in profile.

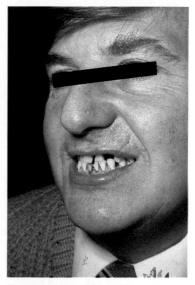

Fig. 136 Acromegaly. Prognathism—note over-riding lower teeth.

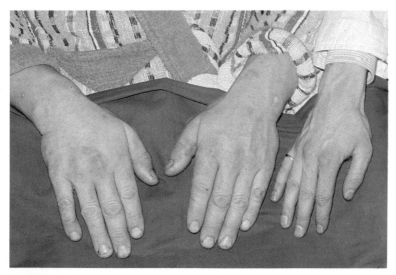

Fig. 137 Acromegaly. Large spade-like hands of patient, compared with a normal hand.

Thyroid disorders

Hypothyroidism

Patients with deficiency of thyroid hormone may develop a constellation of rheumatic manifestations. The typical facies (Figs 138 & 139) will often alert diagnostic suspicion, but sometimes general clinical features are more masked. The principal rheumatic syndromes associated with hypothyroidism are:

- Pain and stiffness in proximal muscles.
- Polyarthritis: bilateral and symmetrical. Usually affects knees, often wrists, MCP or MTP joints, and occasionally ankles and elbows. This is an inflammatory arthropathy, although there may be superimposed osteoarthrosis.
- Monarthritis associated with osteolytic lesions, usually in children.
- Carpal tunnel syndrome.
- Secondary gout.
- Pains in neck, shoulders and upper chest in about 10% of patients with Hashimoto's thyroiditis.

Hyperthyroidism

Hyperthyroidism (appearance shown in Figs 140 & 141) is not a cause of arthritis, but rheumatic manifestations may occur:

- Myopathy affecting proximal muscles and associated with weakness and cramp.
- Thyroid acropachy. This affects about 1% of hyperthyroid patients and is characterized by soft-tissue swelling of fingers and toes, digital clubbing, pretibial myxoedema and exophthalmos. It follows successful treatment of hyperthyroidism.

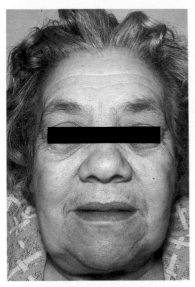

Fig. 138 Hypothyroidism. Typical myxoedema facies in female patient.

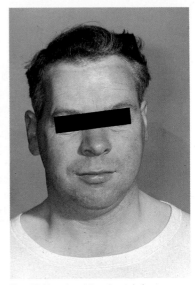

Fig. 139 Hypothyroidism. Less obvious myxoedema facies in male patient.

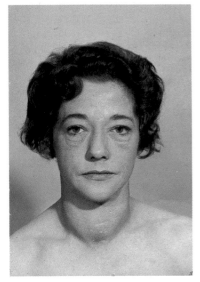

Fig. 140 Hyperthyroidism. Note goitre. Otherwise appearance normal.

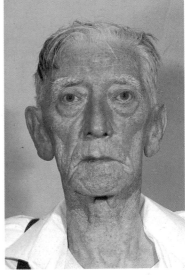

Fig. 141 Hyperthyroidism. Note lean face and bright, slightly prominent eyes. Goitre not obvious.

Adrenal disorders

Addison's
disease

A condition due to *hypoactivity* of the adrenal cortex (named after T. Addison, 1793–1860). Although not responsible for rheumatic features, its therapy may be. Figure 142 shows an Addisonian patient treated with corticosteroids which, in excess or on withdrawal, may give rise to musculoskeletal pain.

Cushing's
syndrome

A condition due to *hyperactivity* of the adrenal cortex (named after H. Cushing 1869–1939). Identical features may develop to those seen with long-term, high-dose corticosteroid therapy. In addition to the superficial stigmata of the syndrome (Figs 143 & 144), patients may develop the following:

- Profound osteoporosis, resulting in crush fractures of vertebral bodies with wedging and severe back pain.
- Avascular necrosis of the femoral or humeral head.
- Rheumatic manifestations due to 'general' features of the disease (e.g. muscle wasting) and to rheumatic features of 'complications' (e.g. diabetes mellitus).
- Although poorly documented, it might be expected that inadequate replacement therapy after surgical treatment might give rise to the steroid-withdrawal rheumatic syndrome of intense arthralgia, joint tenderness and periarticular oedema.

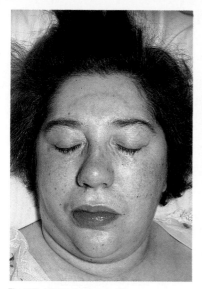

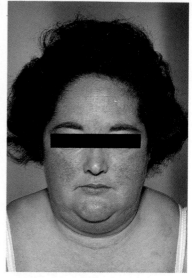

Fig. 142 Addison's disease. Note pigmentation across forehead. Cushingoid facies from steroid therapy.

Fig. 143 Cushing's syndrome. Pre-operative facies in patient with adrenal adenoma.

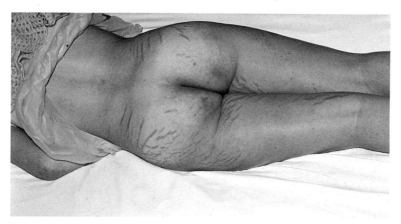

Fig. 144 Iatrogenic hypercorticism. Striae atrophicae due to steroid therapy for RA.

25 / **Neurological disorders**

Syringomyelia

Definition The presence of cavities (Greek, *syrinx* = tube or pipe) surrounded by gliosis near the central canal of the spinal cord and medulla.

Prevalence Age of onset: 10–60 yr; usually 25–40 yr. M:F = 3:1.

Aetiology Probably based on a congenital abnormality with abnormal closure of the embryonic spinal canal and secondary gliosis of the cavities thus formed.

Clinical features The onset is very insidious. Wasting and weakness of the small muscles of the hand are the commonest early symptoms. Sensory or trophic lesions may be the first to attract attention. These patients are sometimes referred to rheumatologists in the mistaken belief that the diagnosis is 'arthritis'. The features giving rise to erroneous diagnosis include: finger contractures (Figs 145 & 146), digital mutilation (Fig. 147) and limitation of joint motion and power (Fig. 148).

Radiological features Trophic changes of terminal phalanges may suggest scleroderma, psoriatic arthritis or polvinylchloride disease. Charcot's arthropathy may be present—about 25% having this feature (see p. 89).

Laboratory features Unhelpful.

Management
- Irradiation of the affected region of the spinal cord and medulla.
- Treatment of Charcot's joints (see page 89).
- Physiotherapy to improve muscle power.
- Local treatment for trophic skin changes.
- Avoidance of further trauma.

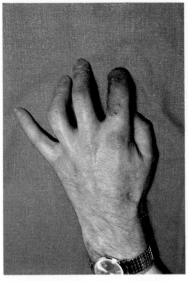

Fig. 145 Syringomyelia. 'Main en griffe' and cigarette-burn scars.

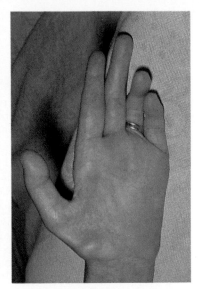

Fig. 146 Syringomyelia. 'Benediction hand'—note muscle wasting and associated prominent thumb CM joint.

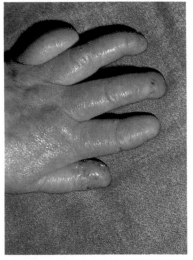

Fig. 147 Syringomyelia. Mutilated, fleshy ('main succulente') and scarred hand.

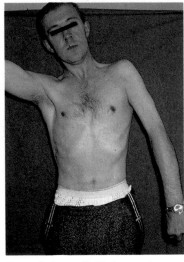

Fig. 148 Syringomyelia. Weakness and wasting with severely limited abduction.

Charcot's arthropathy

Definition A condition characterized by marked disorganisation of a joint and destruction of joint surfaces, associated with diminished pain sensation. Named after J. M. Charcot (1825–93).

Prevalence Depends on cause but, in general, this is an uncommon disorder. M:F = 3:2. Usually after middle age, but may be seen in children with congenital lesions.

Aetiology The most common predisposing disorders are tabes dorsalis, diabetes mellitus and syringomyelia. Rarer causes include hereditary sensory radicular neuropathy and Charcot–Marie–Tooth disease; congenital indifference to pain; spinal cord disease and peripheral nerve lesions; familial dysautonomia.

Clinical features Pain may be present initially, but it is often absent or diminished in later stages. Monarticular in 70%—often the knee.
Acute stage: warm, tender and swollen joint.
Chronic stage: swelling, instability, crepitus and grotesque deformity (Figs 149 & 150).

Radiological features These include sclerosis of bone ends; realignment and remodelling; loss of joint space; loose bodies; massive osteophytes; periarticular calcification and fractures. Most of these features are shown in Figure 151.

Laboratory features Unhelpful.

Management Rest is important in acute stage, and avoidance of trauma. Later: stabilization with appliances to prevent or correct deformity. Consider arthrodesis, but bear in mind that non-union may occur.

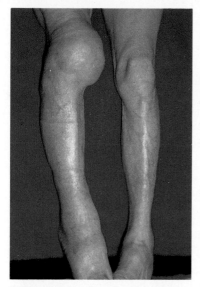

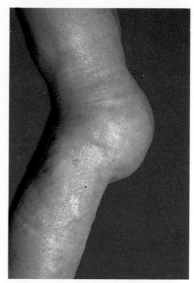

Fig. 149 Charcot's arthropathy. Charcot knee with secondary arthritis of ankle and foot.

Fig. 150 Charcot's arthropathy. Detail of above. Note deformity and marks from supporting bandage.

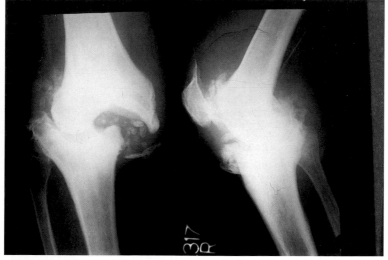

Fig. 151 Charcot's arthropathy. Gross destruction and degeneration, and loose bodies (AP and lateral views).

Carpal tunnel syndrome

Caused by compression of the median nerve at the wrist, this is the most common of the 'entrapment neuropathies'. It occurs in adults of all ages, particularly in women. It may be idiopathic or associated with various general disorders, e.g. obesity, pregnancy, myxoedema, acromegaly, rheumatoid arthritis and osteoarthrosis. The features of pain and muscle wasting may be mistaken for the results of joint disease, as may the relative prominence of wrist and thumb bones due to muscle wasting (Fig. 152).

Herpes zoster

Infection of the posterior root ganglion with the varicella virus, causing segmental pain and a vesicular rash (Fig. 153). It may be associated with two types of rheumatic disorder:

- Arthritis of the small joints of the hand in the distribution of affected nerves.
- Shoulder–hand syndrome. The painful pre-rash stage may suggest arthritis of peripheral or spinal joints.

Polyneuropathy

This is of rheumatological relevance for two reasons:

- If due to a purely neurological disorder, the symptoms (pain, paraesthesiae) and signs (motor and/or sensory deficit) may suggest a rheumatic disorder.
- It may be an established complication of a chronic rheumatic disorder (e.g. RA, SLE). Clinical signs, such as the one shown in Figure 154, will clarify the significance of the neuropathy; in this case toxic polyneuropathy due to lead poisoning manifested by the classical blue line on the gums.

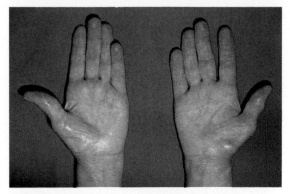

Fig. 152 Carpal tunnel syndrome. Right thenar wasting with prominence of CM joint.

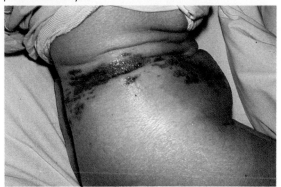

Fig. 153 Herpes zoster. Eruption localized to right T9 dermatome.

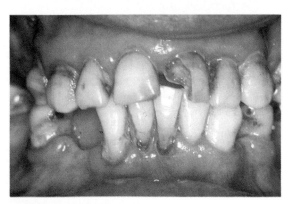

Fig. 154 Lead poisoning. Typical blue line at upper and lower gingival margins.

Neuralgic amyotrophy

A condition characterized by pain in the shoulder, which may be mistaken for the shoulder–hand syndrome or frozen shoulder. It is more common in men (M:F = 2:1). There is a history of preceding illness, operation or trauma in 50%.

Clinical features   Main features: sudden pain in shoulder, followed by limited movement and, later, nerve palsy. The neurological deficit, most often serratus anterior paralysis (Fig. 155), recovers slowly over 12–18 months and does not recur.

Management   Analgesics and physiotherapy.

Neurofibromatosis

This hereditary disease (von Recklinghausen's disease, after F. D. von Recklinghausen 1833–1910) is characterized by multiple neuromas or neurofibromas (Fig. 156), pigmented skin lesions and neurological manifestations due to involvement of nerve trunks, nerve roots and spinal cord. Skeletal manifestations include kyphoscoliosis, hyperostosis of facial bones, enlargement of the calvarium, and hyperostosis and curvature of long bones.

Intracranial tumour

As with stroke syndromes, this may enter into rheumatological differential diagnosis (Fig. 157). Cerebral changes may be confused with antirheumatic drug effects or the psychological and psychiatric manifestations of systemic rheumatoses (e.g. SLE). Weakness and deformity in limbs may be ascribed to concomitant arthritis, particularly in the elderly.

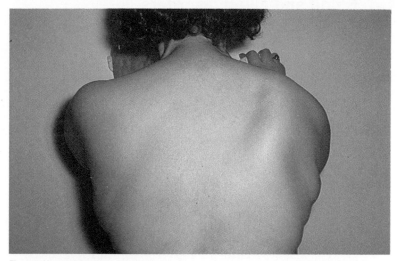

Fig. 155 Neuralgic amyotrophy. Winging of right scapula due to paralysis of serratus anterior.

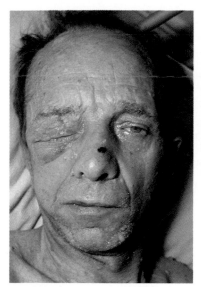

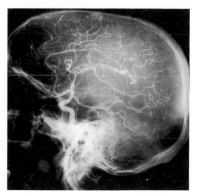

Fig. 157 Intracranial tumour.

Fig. 156 Neurofibromatosis. Plexiform neuroma affecting right eye and cutaneous fibromata.

26 / Blood and allied disorders

Haemorrhagic disorders

The main rheumatological impact of haemorrhagic and related disorders is blood in the joint—haemarthrosis. This may occur in various conditions, including primary synovial sarcomata, pigmented villonodular synovitis, osteoarthrosis, rheumatoid arthritis, pseudogout, after trauma, as well as in primary haematological disorders (notably haemophilia).

Clinical features The physical signs of a hot, tender joint with or without surface manifestations of periarticular haematoma are similar whatever the cause. The patient shown in Figure 158 had RA, but the appearance would be similar in haemophilia.Scurvy has been included here (Fig. 159) as massive ecchymoses may occur (particularly in adults) near joints but not in them. (These patients may also develop arthritis.)

Haemoglobinopathies

Certain haemoglobinopathies, particularly sickle-cell disease, may be associated with rheumatological features. In sickle-cell disease it is the homozygotes who develop arthritis due to bone infarcts resulting from thrombotic crises. This also occurs in sickle-cell and β thalassaemia, in addition to the typical clinical (Fig. 160) and laboratory features of haemoglobinopathies.

Radiological features The main radiological signs are areas of porosis or sclerosis representing infarcts; dactylitis due to periosteal proliferation; evidence of bone marrow hyperplasia in the skull ('hair-on-end' appearance), spine ('cupped' vertebrae, Fig. 161), and long bones near joints (cortical thinning and widening of medulla); avascular necrosis and salmonella osteomyelitis.

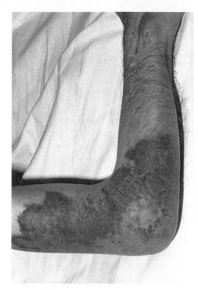

Fig. 158 Haemorrhagic disorders. Haemarthrosis with periarticular haematoma in RA.

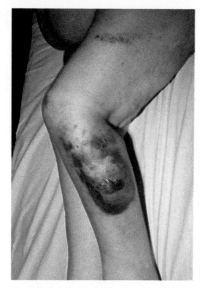

Fig. 159 Haemorrhagic disorders. Massive ecchymosis due to scurvy.

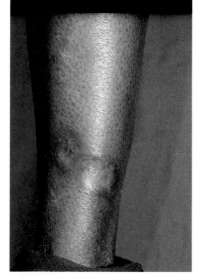

Fig. 160 Haemoglobinopathies. Leg scars in sickle-cell disease.

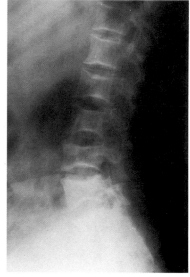

Fig. 161 Haemoglobinopathies. Spondylopathy in sickle-cell disease. Note cupped vertebrae.

27 / Diseases of the digestive system

Upper GI tract   Conditions of rheumatological significance are: aphthous ulcers (e.g. Behçet's syndrome, ulcerative colitis), oesophagitis (e.g. drug therapy), peptic symptoms or ulceration (e.g. drugs (Fig. 162), underlying neoplasia), chronic inflammatory small bowel disease (e.g. Crohn's disease, Whipple's disease), malabsorption due to rheumatoid-induced amyloidosis and infarction due to RA.

Lower GI tract   Conditions of rheumatological significance are: ulcerative colitis (Fig. 163); Crohn's colitis, Behçet's syndrome, Reiter's disease, shigellosis, colonic and rectal neoplasms.

Liver   Liver disease (often little more than altered liver function, without histological changes) is seen in RA and its variants (e.g. Felty's syndrome and Sjögren's syndrome). SLE may be associated with occasional perihepatitis. Unrelated to SLE, chronic active hepatitis with LE cells ('lupoid hepatitis') may be associated with an arthritis simulating RA. Hepatic involvement may be a prominent feature in certain malignant disorders (Fig. 164) having rheumatic accompaniments.

Pancreas   Acute pancreatitis, chronic relapsing pancreatitis and pancreatic carcinoma may be associated with transient polyarthritis, accompanied by tender nodular skin lesions due to subcutaneous fat necrosis. The arthritis is usually synchronous with the skin lesions but may precede them and other manifestations of pancreatic disease by several weeks. Apart from biochemical tests, the plain abdominal X-ray may give valuable clues concerning the presence of pancreatic disease. Note pancreatic calcification in Figure 165.

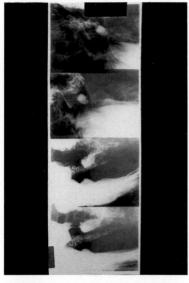

Fig. 162 Upper GI tract. Barium meal showing gastric ulcer, probably steroid-induced.

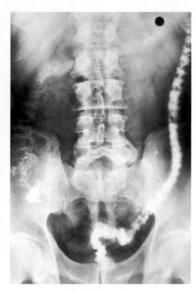

Fig. 163 Lower GI tract. Barium enema showing colitis on left (right normal).

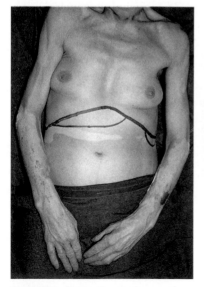

Fig. 164 Liver disease. Hepatosplenomegaly. (This patient had Hodgkin's disease)

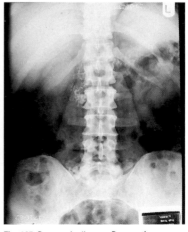

Fig. 165 Pancreatic disease. Pancreatic calcification in chronic active pancreatitis.

28 / Diseases of the urinary system

General comment
Diseases of the urinary system, principally of the kidneys, may be associated with a multitude of rheumatic ailments. The renal–rheumatic association may occur as part of a systemic connective tissue disorder (e.g. SLE), as part of a nephrotoxic syndrome (e.g. analgesic nephropathy), or as the musculoskeletal manifestations of chronic renal failure, dialysis or transplantation.

Clinical features
The musculoskeletal features of renal disease include the following: secondary hyperparathyroidism, osteomalacia, calcium pyrophosphate arthropathy (pseudogout), extraskeletal calcification, acute gouty arthritis, monarticular crystal-negative arthritis, polyarticular crystal-negative arthritis and septic arthritis.

Apart from osteoarticular manifestations, the usual general stigmata of acute and chronic renal disease should be sought. Naked-eye examination of the urine is an integral part of the clinical examination (Figs 166 & 167).

Radiological features
These may be divided into those relevant to osteoarticular manifestations (covered elsewhere in this book under appropriate sections), and those concerning examination of the urinary tract. The value of the plain abdominal X-ray (Fig. 168) should not be underrated, although more detailed examination by means of contrast radiography (Fig. 169) will be necessary in most patients.

Management
This is according to the specific nature of the osteoarticular problem (see appropriate section) and the type of urinary tract problem.

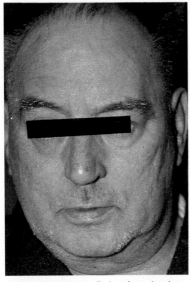

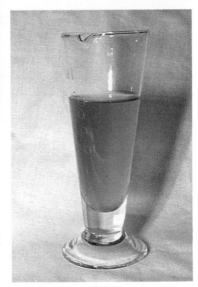

Fig. 166 Renal disease. Facies of a patient in chronic renal failure.

Fig. 167 Renal disease. Haematuria.

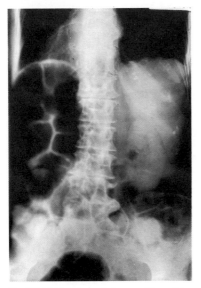

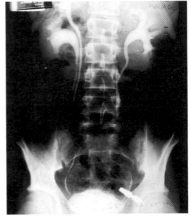

Fig. 169 IVP. Duplex right kidney and ureter (with hydronephrosis).

Fig. 168 Plain radiograph. Can provide useful information. Normal left renal shadow; right obscured.

29 / **Hypercholesterolaemia**

Definition An hereditary disorder of cholesterol metabolism characterized in homozygotes by a markedly raised plasma cholesterol, xanthomatosis and premature atherosclerosis. It may be associated with arthritis.

Prevalence Rare. M = F. Age of onset: 5–10 yr.

Aetiology Autosomal intermediate transmission.

Clinical features Half of the homozygotes develop arthritis. Onset is acute, often migratory, affecting large joints—usually knees. Cholesterol deposits present as unilateral (Fig. 170) or bilateral (Fig. 171) xanthelasma. Xanthomata are seen at other sites, e.g. elbows (Fig. 172) and in relation to tendons and periosteum. Other features include corneal arcus, premature atherosclerosis and cardiac murmurs.

Radiological features The joints are usually normal. There may be phalangeal erosions not involving joint surface.

Laboratory features Raised plasma cholesterol; ESR raised in attacks of arthritis.

Management **Symptomatic:** salicylates.
Diet: low cholesterol and high polyunsaturated fat diet. Cholestyramine.

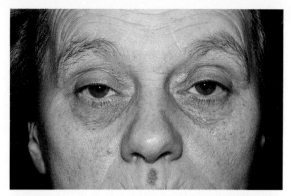

Fig. 170 Hypercholesterolaemia. Unilateral xanthelasma palpebrarum.

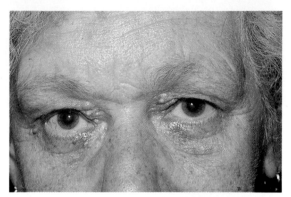

Fig. 171 Hypercholesterolaemia. Bilateral xanthelasma palpebrarum.

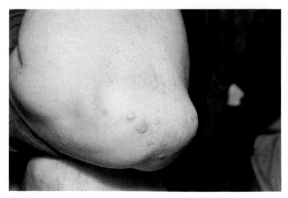

Fig. 172 Hypercholesterolaemia. Xanthomata on elbow.

30 / Sarcoidosis

Definition	A condition of unknown aetiology characterized by multisystem involvement due to granulomatous inflammation, particularly affecting lymph nodes, spleen, liver and lungs. There may be an associated arthritis, and the details below concern this (as opposed to the parent disorder).
Prevalence	F:M = 3:1. Age of onset: 15–50 yr; peak 20–30 yr. It affects about 10% of patients with sarcoidosis.
Aetiology	Both the cause and mechanism of this disease are unknown, but many theories have been proposed, mainly based on hypersensitivity.
Clinical features	Arthritis of sarcoidosis of two types: • Early acute transient type. This often affects wrists (Fig. 173), elbows (Fig. 174), shoulders, MCP and PIP joints. Rarely big toe—resembling gout. • Chronic persistent type.
Radiological features	The joints are usually normal. Cystic changes are occasionally seen in hands or feet. Chest X-ray shows hilar lymphadenopathy (Fig. 175) in 75% and/or pulmonary infiltration (50%).
Laboratory features	Raised ESR. Tests for rheumatoid factor are positive in 10%. Hypergammaglobulinaemia is seen in 10%. Mantoux is negative in 70%; Kveim test is positive in 70%. Synovial biopsy or biopsy of other tissues—granulomata and inflammatory changes.
Management	Analgesic/anti-inflammatory drugs; steroids for severe 'resistant' arthritis or for other indications (e.g. iritis, hypercalcaemia).

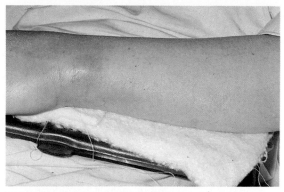

Fig. 173 Sarcoidosis. Acute arthritis of wrist. Note shiny erythema overlying joint.

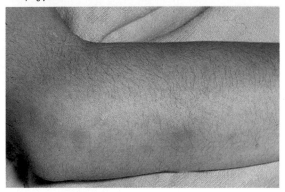

Fig. 174 Sarcoidosis. Acute arthritis of elbow and erythema nodosum on forearm.

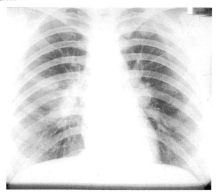

Fig. 175 Sarcoidosis. Bilateral hilar lymphadenopathy.

31 / Toxic erythemas

Erythema nodosum

An acute self-limiting disorder characterized by an eruption consisting of painful and tender nodules in the skin on the front of the legs (Fig. 176) and back of the forearms (Fig. 177). The lesions are at first bright red, later darker, and eventually fade like bruises. The acute illness may be accompanied by malaise, fever, joint pain and swelling (note arthrocentesis site Fig. 176). Associated conditions include sarcoidosis (commonest cause in UK—35% of all cases); various infections, particularly streptococcosis and primary tuberculosis; ulcerative colitis, Crohn's disease, Behçet's syndrome; malignant disease; drug sensitivities, e.g. to sulphonamides; idiopathic—10%.

Treatment: rest and aspirin or other NSAIDs.

Erythema multiforme

An eruption consisting of circular or irregular erythematous blotches. These are often 'target' or 'iris' lesions (Fig. 178). The rash commonly occurs on the backs of hands and forearms. Polyarthritis is an uncommon complication. It often follows drug therapy or vaccination. Often no cause is found. No specific treatment available. Antibiotics may be needed to control secondary infection of eye or mucosal lesions. Systemic steroids may be required for severe bullous or mucosal types.

Other erythemas

Erythema marginatum has been mentioned under rheumatic fever. Generalized erythema, having scarlatiform, morbilliform, macular of circinate features, may be associated with drug therapy, other dermatoses or infections (e.g. syphilis), all of which may be accompanied directly or indirectly by joint involvement.

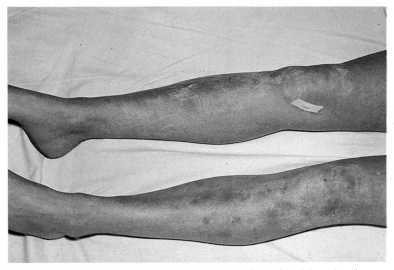

Fig. 176 Erythema nodosum. Rash on both legs and synovitis of knees (right joint aspirated).

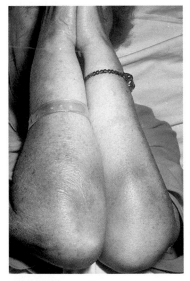

Fig. 177 Erythema nodosum. Rash on both forearms. Site infrequent but appearance of lesions typical.

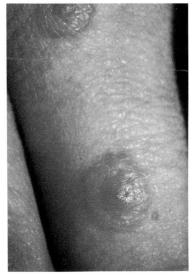

Fig. 178 Erythema multiforme. Typical 'target' lesions.

32 / **Osteoporosis**

Definition	Osteoporotic bone is normal in composition but reduced in amount—skeletal atrophy or osteopenia.
Prevalence	Depends on cause. The commonest types are post-menopausal and 'senile' osteoporosis.
Aetiology	***Idiopathic:*** post-menopausal, 'senile' (or elderly), pregnancy, young adult, juvenile. ***Known or postulated:*** immobilization, endocrine, chromosomal (Turner's syndrome), with osteomalacia and others (including RA, osteogenesis imperfecta).
Clinical features	These include localized pain, deformity and fracture. The commonest deformity is loss of height due to vertebral collapse ('shrinkage' in old people is due to osteoporosis). Examination may reveal loss of trunk height, a transverse abdominal crease and kyphosis (Fig. 179).
Radiological features	Before structural collapse, porotic changes become evident (Fig. 180). Vertical trabeculae become more prominent due to loss of horizontal trabeculae. Irregular wedging of vertebrae (Fig. 181), without the prominent 'cod-fish spine', due to vertebral concavity is seen in osteomalacia (except in the young or in inherited osteoporosis).
Laboratory features	Plasma and urine values are within the normal range. Biopsy is sometimes done to exclude other disorders (e.g. osteomalacia, leukaemia, myeloma).
Management	Exercise and exercises. Avoid immobility, and jolts and other sources of injury. Mechanical supports (braces) may be necessary. Oral calcium supplements, vitamin D, fluoride, anabolic steroids, calcitonin and parathormone have been tried, but evidence is conflicting. The most convincing treatment is oestrogen therapy in post-menopausal women.

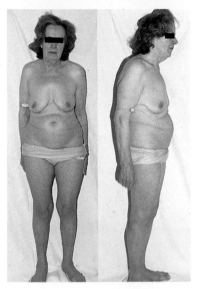

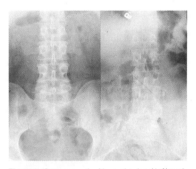

Fig. 179 Osteoporosis. Loss of trunk height and transverse abdominal crease (*left*). Kyphosis (*right*).

Fig. 180 Osteoporosis. Normal spine (*left*) and porotic spine (*right*).

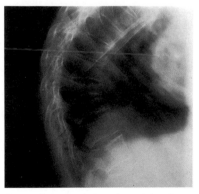

Fig. 181 Osteoporosis. Irregular wedging of vertebrae.

33 / Osteomalacia and rickets

Definition — Difficult to define. There is defective mineralization of organic bone matrix. It is seen histologically in undecalcified bone as an excess of osteoid. Rickets is the childhood disorder; osteomalacia is the adult counterpart.

Prevalence — Depends on cause. The condition is becoming more prevalent in the UK since increase in Asian population.

Aetiology — Causes are vitamin D deficiency, malabsorption, renal disease and other disorders (e.g. anticonvulsant osteomalacia, tumour rickets, vitamin D-dependent rickets).

Clinical features — The main symptoms are bone pain, deformity, tenderness and weakness of proximal muscles. Deformity is most marked during childhood (bowing of long bones, 'rickety rosary', Harrison's sulcus and bossing of frontal and parietal bones). Clinical features are also seen from underlying disorder (e.g. renal failure, malabsorption).

Radiological features — In rickets the characteristic features are widening of the growth plate and of the metaphysis, which is cupped and ragged. In osteomalacia the classical sign is the Looser's zone (after E. Looser, 1877–1936). This is the radiological hallmark of active osteomalacia and appears as a ribbon-like area of demineralisation (Figs 182 & 183). The vertebral bodies are porotic and uniformly biconcave (Fig. 184A: 'cod-fish spine'). When parathyroid activity is prominent the 'rugger-jersey spine' (Fig. 184B) may be a feature due to increased density of end plates.

Laboratory features — Histology (see above); total plasma calcium low or normal; inorganic phosphate low; alkaline phosphatase usually increased. Urinary calcium is low; urinary phosphate is increased.

Management — Vitamin D. Treatment of underlying disorder.

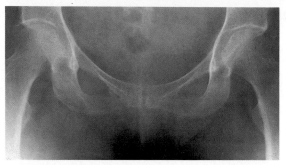

Fig. 182 Pelvic Looser's zones.

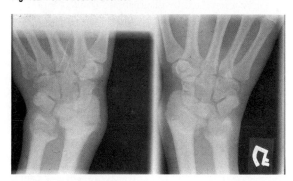

Fig. 183 Looser's zones in forearm bones.

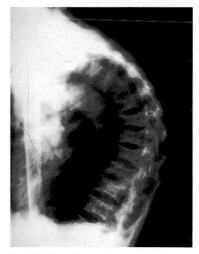

Fig. 184A 'Cod-fish spine'.

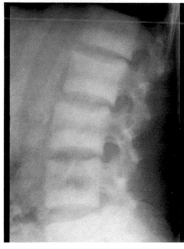

Fig. 184B 'Rugger-jersey spine.'

34 / Paget's disease of bone

Definition   A disorder of unknown aetiology (named after J. Paget 1814–99) affecting one or more bones, particularly the pelvis, femur, skull, tibia and vertebrae.

Prevalence   Rare before age 30 yr; 0.5% at 40 yr; 10% at 90 yr. M:F = 2:1. In the UK about 650 000 have Paget's disease (but only 5% with symptoms).

Aetiology   The cause not known but the pathophysiology is characterized by disorganised overactivity of bone, with parallel activities of rapid resorption and rapid laying 'down of new bone.

Clinical features   Mainly bone pain and deformities. Four types of arthritis may occur: arthritis due to disease adjacent to joint; calcific periarthritis; acute gout and spondylopathy simulating spondylitis. Characteristic features include large skull (Fig. 185), bowed tibia (Fig. 186), deafness and kyphosis. Rarer features include spinal cord, nerve root or cauda equina compression, high output cardiac failure, and osteogenic sarcoma.

Radiological features   Typical features of this 'busy-bone' disorder are shown in Fig. 187. Note the 'fluffy' appearance of pagetic bone. Note also the coarse trabeculation and expansion and thickening of affected bones. The disease does not cross joint lines.

Laboratory features   Alkaline phosphatase is usually raised. Plasma calcium is usually normal; plasma phosphate may be in upper normal range. Urinary total hydroxyproline is increased. Bone biopsy is required only rarely to confirm diagnosis or exclude malignant disease.

Management   Analgesics; 'specific' treatment with calcitonin, mithramycin or EHDP; treatment of complications (e.g. fractures, cardiac failure, osteogenic sarcoma).

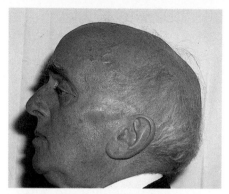

Fig. 185 Paget's disease. Enlarged skull.

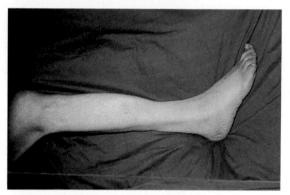

Fig. 186 Paget's disease. Mid-shaft bowing of tibia ('sabre tibia').

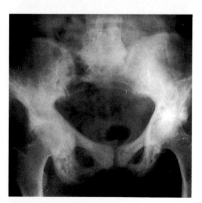

Fig. 187 Paget's disease. Typical changes. Note hip joint line not crossed.

35 / Hyperparathyroidism

Definition	Excessive formation of parathormone usually by an autonomous parathyroid adenoma (rarely hyperplasia or carcinoma).
Prevalence	Present in 3–10% of patients with recurrent renal calculi. F:M = 5:1. Age of onset: 30–70 yr.
Aetiology	This can be explained in terms of the main effects of parathormone which are: to reduce reabsorption of phosphate, to stimulate osteoclastic bone resorption, to stimulate renal reabsorption of calcium and calcium absorption across the small intestine.
Clinical features	Arthritis is a rare presenting feature. It may follow parathyroidectomy. The main types of arthritis in this disorder are:

- Osteogenic synovitis due to softening and collapse of subchondral bone, arthritis occurring for same reason as in osteomalacia.
- Pseudogout due to hypercalcaemia.
- Gout due to diminished tubular uric acid secretion.

Non-rheumatological features include:

- Anorexia, vomiting and constipation.
- Polyuria, polydypsia and renal colic.
- Weakness and tiredness.
- Band keratopathy.
- Mental changes.

Radiological features	Subperiosteal reabsorption of the phalanges (Fig. 188) is diagnostic. It is thought to occur more markedly on the radial border of the proximal and middle phalanges of the index and middle fingers (Fig. 189). Resorption and shortening may affect the distal phalanges (Figs 188 & 189) but is not pathognomonic (it also occurs in polyvinylchloride workers' disease, scleroderma and psoriatic arthritis).

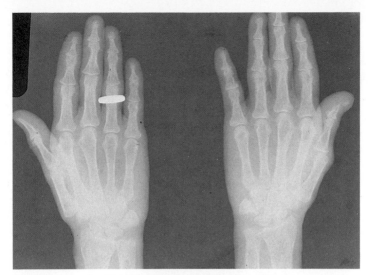

Fig. 188 Hyperparathyroidism. Distribution of subperiosteal erosions and acro-osteolysis.

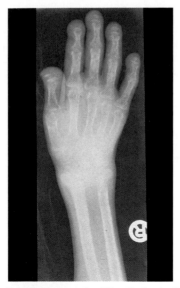

Fig. 189 Hyperparathyroidism. Further details of subperiosteal erosions and acro-osteolysis.

Radiological features (contd)

Resorption may also occur in the medial borders of the upper tibiae, symphysis pubis, femoral necks and outer ends of clavicles. Occasionally more localized lesions are seen. These include 'cysts' in the ribs or other bones and a 'pepper-pot' appearance in the skull. Cortical resorption and trabecular coarsening may also give the skull a Paget's-like appearance (Fig. 190). The spine may show the 'rugger-jersey' effect (Fig. 191), but this is of little diagnostic value. Soft-tissue calcification may be present (Fig. 191).

Laboratory features

- Raised serum calcium, low phosphate.
- Alkaline phosphatase may be increased, but is normal if there is no clinical or radiological evidence of bone disease (the majority).
- Raised urea in later stages.
- Hyperuricaemia in 50%.
- ESR normal.
- Tests for rheumatoid factor negative.

Management

Orthodox teaching is that the only treatment for primary hyperparathyroidism is surgical. However, conservative management is reasonable for asymptomatic patients with mild hypercalcaemia (> 3 mmol/l). The operation should involve removing the adenoma together with identification and examination of the remaining three glands (10% have multiple adenomata).

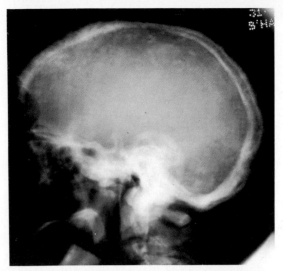

Fig. 190 Hyperparathyroidism. Typical features in skull due to cortical resorption and trabecular coarsening.

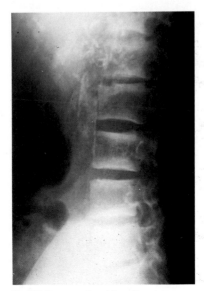

Fig. 191 Hyperparathyroidism. 'Rugger-jersey spine'. Also note aortic calcification.

36 / Avascular (ischaemic) necrosis

Definition and aetiology	Bone necrosis usually due to interference to the blood supply. This may be due to arteritis, external vascular pressure, trauma, thrombosis or embolism. Clinical subdivisions of avascular necrosis are: traumatic, secondary to existing arthropathies, secondary to systemic conditions and idiopathic.
Prevalence	May occur at any age, in either sex, depending on the underlying cause.
Clinical features	Usually one or both hips are affected, though rarely knees or shoulders. The condition is bilateral in 30%. Features of underlying disease are present, if there is one.
Radiological features	Examples of early (Fig. 192) and later (Fig. 193) avascular necrosis, due to RA, are shown here. The main radiological stages can be summarized as follows:

- A crescentic area of rarefaction of subchondral bone.
- Irregularity or flattening of the affected epiphyses, or a depressed segment of subchondral bone.
- An area of porosis, or patchy sclerosis, which in the hip joint appears as a sector of the femoral head.
- Separation of necrotic fragments, particularly in the knee, and collapse of bone underlying the sector of affected joint surface.
- Complete joint destruction, or disappearance of the femoral or humeral heads.

Laboratory features	Unhelpful.
Management	Best without weight-bearing; this sometimes allows healing and remodelling. Surgical treatment with arthroplasty is often required when the joint becomes severely deformed.

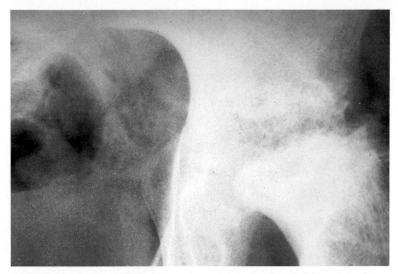

Fig. 192 Avascular nercrosis. Relatively recent destructive changes. Note 'fluffy' irregularity of femoral head.

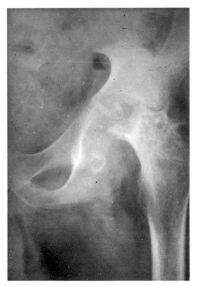

Fig. 193 Avascular necrosis. Long-standing destructive changes. Note well-defined margin of pseudoarthrosis.

37 / Ankylosing hyperostosis (Forestier's disease)

Definition Also known as Zuckergusswirbelsaüle, hyperostotic spondylosis, vertebral melorheostosis, Forestier's or Baastrup's disease. This is a condition of the elderly in which there is exuberant bony outgrowth from the spine.

Prevalence Most commonly seen in men over age 50.
Frequency: 14% in males and 5% in females over age 35.

Aetiology Some regard it as a variant of spondylosis but it is probably a separate entity. It has been attributed to increased growth hormone output, but little is known about its aetiology, and no family surveys have been recorded.

Clinical features The condition is often asymptomatic. Sometimes stiffness is present without pain. Examination may reveal a slight restriction of spinal movement, but this is not of spondylitic pattern. There are no postural changes, and peripheral joint involvement is not a feature. Diabetes mellitus is often associated.

Radiological features Typical patterns of ossification are shown in Figures 194–196. Characteristically, the layer of ossification extends throughout the entire height of some vertebrae (Fig. 196). The ossified protuberances may extend upwards as 'candle-flame' lesions or downward as 'dripping candle-wax'. The apophyseal joints and the sacroiliac joints (Fig. 197) are normal, distinguishing the disorder from ankylosing spondylitis.

Laboratory features ESR is normal. Calcium, phosphate and alkaline phosphatase are normal. HLA B27 and rheumatoid factor are negative.

Management Urine and blood tests may reveal diabetes mellitus. Management also involves symptomatic treatment and maintenance of mobility.

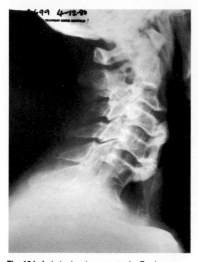

Fig. 194 Ankylosing hyperostosis. Exuberant flamed-shape exostoses over front of cervical vertebrae.

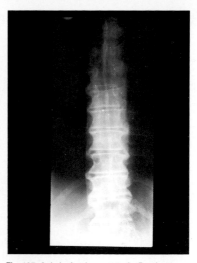

Fig. 195 Ankylosing hyperostosis. Bamboo-like thoracic spine due to thick bands of paravertebral ossification.

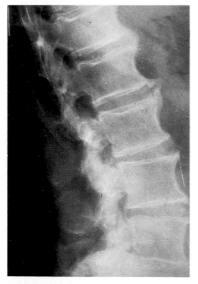

Fig. 196 Ankylosing hyperostosis. 'Candle-wax' (or 'sugar-icing') ossification throughout upper lumbar vertebrae.

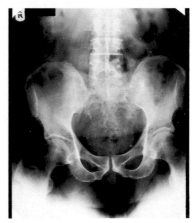

Fig. 197 Ankylosing hyperostosis. Pelvic exostoses. Note patency of sacroiliac joints.

38 / Marfan's syndrome

Definition An inherited disorder characterized by skeletal deformity, arachnodactyly, dislocated lenses and aortic dilatation (named after A. B-J. Marfan 1858–1942).

Prevalence Rare—estimated at 1.5 per 1 000 000 of the population.

Aetiology Autosomal dominant inheritance with wide variability of expression.

Clinical and radiological features Excessive lengthening of the digits, or arachnodactyly (Fig. 198), is one of the cardinal features, although it is not pathognomonic. The tall asthenic build and 'El Greco' facies are also characteristic (Fig. 199), although non-asthenic forms do exist. Disproportionately long extremities (Fig. 200), a high palate, thoracic asymmetry and articular hypermobility are other typical skeletal features. About 50% have eye defects, most commonly ectopia lentis, and 20% have cardiovascular anomalies, including septal defects, conduction defects and aneuryms. Later manifestations are aortic incompetence and dissecting aneurysm. Backache occurs in 30%, and 20% have peripheral arthritis.

Laboratory features In the urine, homocystine is absent (cf. homocystinuria which may resemble Marfan's syndrome), and hydroxyproline may be increased.

Management Treatment of aortic valve disease (the main cause of death) is essential. Other features requiring treatment include scoliosis and excessive growth, especially in girls. This has been achieved by an oestrogen–progesterone regime.

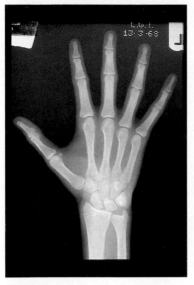

Fig. 198 Marfan's syndrome. Arachnodactyly. Note long, thin phalanges and metacarpals.

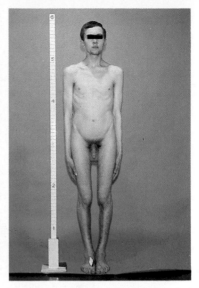

Fig. 199 Marfan's syndrome. Note 'El Greco' facies, pectus excavatum, 'linear' somatype.

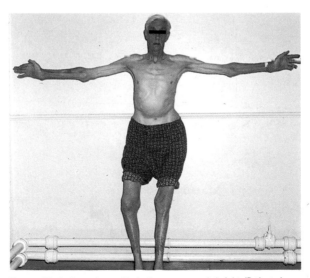

Fig. 200 Marfan's syndrome. Typically, span exceeds height. (Patient also had RA.)

39 / Alkaptonuria

Definition   An hereditary disease caused by a deficiency of the enzyme homogentisic acid oxidase. It is associated with alkaptonuria, the excretion of 'alkaptan' (later identified as homogentisic acid), and ochronosis (*ochros* = sallow), the accumulation of pigment in tissues.

Prevalence   Rare. M:F = 2:1.

Aetiology   Inheritance is by an autosomal recessive character. The lack of homogentisic acid oxidase causes metabolic changes through defective catabolism of phenylalanine and tyrosine.

Clinical features   These include degenerative arthritis of peripheral joints—knees (80%), shoulders (50%) and hips (50%)—and degenerative spondylopathy. The peripheral arthritis clinically resembles osteoarthrosis, and the spinal changes resemble spondylosis. However, if limitation of spinal motion and chest expansion is prominent, the spondylopathy may resemble ankylosing spondylitis. Associated features:

- Black, dark-brown or bluish discoloration of sclera (Fig. 201), cornea, conjunctiva, eyelids and skin, and ear cartilages (Fig. 202). This usually appears in middle age.
- Renal and prostatic calculi.
- Darkening of urine which becomes black on standing or when alkalinized (see p. 125).

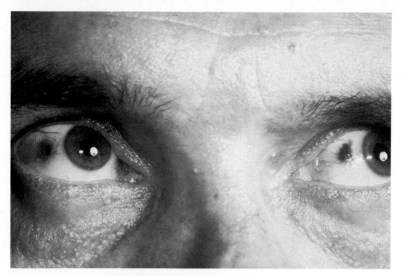

Fig. 201 Alkaptonuria. Patches of ochronotic pigment in sclerae.

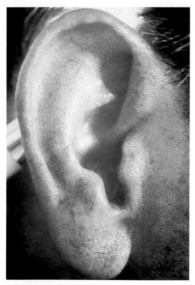

Fig. 202 Alkaptonuria. Ochronotic pigment in lower part of auricular cartilage.

Radiological features

Spine
Dense calcification of intervertebral discs (Fig. 203) is characteristic, indeed pathognomonic. This is associated later with narrowing of disc spaces, sclerosis of adjacent vertebral margins, and, ultimately, disappearance of discs and vertebral fusion (Fig. 204). The sacroiliac joints are normal. There is no ligamentous calcification.

Peripheral joints
Narrowing of joint space is characteristic, with irregularity of joint surface, sclerosis, cystic changes and osteophytes.

Laboratory features

As mentioned before, the urine darkens on standing (Fig. 205) or on alkalinization. When fresh, the urine may be a normal colour. It will give a positive reaction when tested for reducing substances, but not with glucose oxidase. This may lead to an erroneous diagnosis of diabetes mellitus from the use of Benedict's test or Clinitest tablets, or to failure to detect reducing substances if glucose oxidase (Clinistix) is used.

Management

Symptomatic treatment is with analgesics. The logical approach, to reduce homogentisic acid precursors from the diet (e.g. tyrosine or, less specifically, protein), has met with little success.

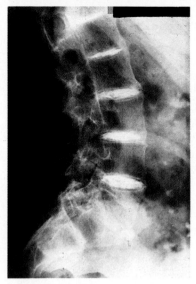

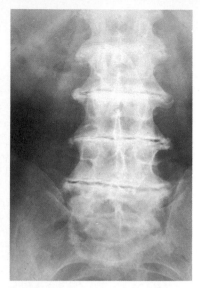

Fig. 203 Alkaptonuria. Intense calcification of intervertebral discs—pathognomic for the disease.

Fig. 204 Alkaptonuria. Marked degenerative changes—intervertebral ossification and disc space narrowing.

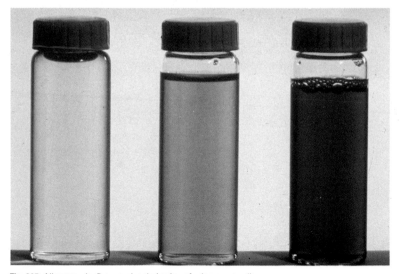

Fig. 205 Alkaptonuria. Progressive darkening of urine on standing.

40 / **Pseudoxanthoma elasticum**

Definition An hereditary disorder caused by a defect in elastic tissue associated with characteristic skin and eye changes, and arterial disease.

Prevalence Rare. Skin lesions are slightly more common in females; angioid streaks are more frequent in males.

Aetiology Inheritance is autosomal recessive, with partial limitation to the female found most often. Irregular dominance has been described.

Clinical features Cutaneous lesions are small, soft chamois-coloured papules parallel to skin lines and folds. This gives rise to a crêpe-like or 'morocco leather' appearance. Another dermal feature is the 'plucked chicken skin' appearance. Sites most often affected are the side of the neck (Fig. 206), axillae, groins, cubital and popliteal fossae, and the periumbilical area. Angioid streaks of the retina are the most characteristic eye lesions and produce the 'tigroid fundus' (Fig. 207). Premature and advanced arterial changes are also common in this disorder. Arthritis is not usually a feature, but intermittent pain, tenderness and swelling of joints have been reported.

Radiological features None of rheumatological significance. (Arthropathy is not destructive).

Laboratory features Biopsy reveals characteristic features—notably calcification in the middle and lower dermis (Fig. 208).

Management Symptomatic treatment for cardiovascular disease. Plastic surgery sometimes helpful to correct cosmetic cutaneous defects.

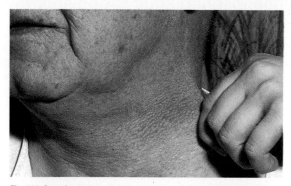

Fig. 206 Pseudoxanthoma elasticum. Typical skin features include the 'plucked chicken skin' appearance seen here at the side of the neck.

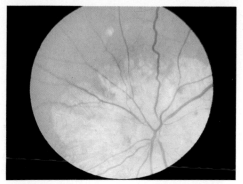

Fig. 207 Pseudoxanthoma elasticum. 'Tigroid fundus'. Note broad, pale, angioid streaks around optic disc.

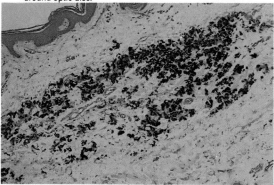

Fig. 208 Pseudoxanthoma elasticum. Calcification in middle and lower dermis.

41 / Hypophosphataemic spondylopathy

Definition   Familial hypophosphataemia is a variant of renal or vitamin D resistant rickets. Childhood rickets heals spontaneously at puberty and is replaced later in life by a spondylitis-like picture—hypophosphataemic spondylopathy.

Prevalence   Rare. F:M = 3:1.

Aetiology   Inheritance is by an X-linked dominant character.

Clinical features   The condition is often more severe in men. Onset is after age 20, sometimes presenting in the elderly. The spine, hips and elbows are commonly affected. Often the shoulders, knees, wrists, ankles, hands and feet are also affected. There is a gradual onset of stiffness, and morning stiffness is slight. Pain is minimal.

Radiological features   The radiological changes include ligamentous calcification, new bone formation and generalized demineralization of bones. This is particularly prominent in the spine (Figs 209 & 210), in and around the pelvis (Fig. 211) and at ligamentous attachments in relation to large joints such as the shoulder (Fig. 212). Obliteration of the sacroiliac joints may occur (see Fig. 211), and this may raise the question of ankylosing spondylitis (in these patients a past history of rickets may be helpful).

Laboratory features   Serum phosphates are low, and serum calcium is low or normal. There is raised alkaline phosphatase. HLA B27 is absent.

Management   Symptomatic: drugs for pain and stiffness, and cautious physiotherapy as there may be demineralization of bones.

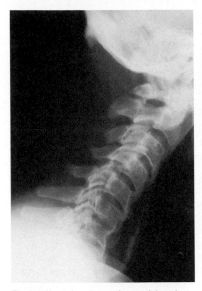

Fig. 209 Hypophosphataemic spondylopathy. Ossification of anterior spinal ligaments of cervical spine.

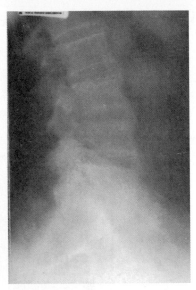

Fig. 210 Hypophosphataemic spondylopathy. Ossification and generalized porosis of lumbar vertebrae.

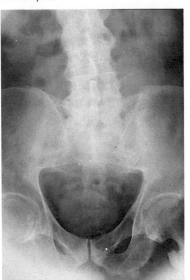

Fig. 211 Hypophosphataemic spondylopathy. Spondylitis-like ossification of pelvis and hips.

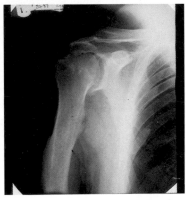

Fig. 212 Hypophosphataemic spondylopathy. Exostoses at muscle attachments around shoulder.

42 / Osteogenesis imperfecta (fragilitas ossium)

Definition Hereditary disease of bone characterized by recurrent fractures and severe deformities.

Prevalence One of the most common of the inherited disorders of the skeleton.

Aetiology Autosomal dominant inheritance, variable in expression. Complete non-penetrance has been reported.

Clinical features Bone fragility is the cardinal feature. This predisposition is variable, some patients experiencing multiple fractures and others few. The fractures heal rapidly, sometimes with residual deformity. A wide bi-temporal diameter and pearly-grey discoloration of the teeth are variable concomitants. Although also variable, blueness of the sclerae (Fig. 213) is a particularly characteristic and classic feature. Figure 214 shows the same feature in an asymptomatic relative. Deafness supervenes in adulthood in about 20%.

Radiological features Fracture(s) is characteristic. Florid callus formation may simulate osteosarcoma. In the 'thick bone' type, the shafts of the long bones are short and wide. In the 'thin bone' type, the diaphyses are gracile.
Undermineralization becomes prominent later in life. The shafts of long bones may become expanded and cystic. The base of the skull may become flattened.

Laboratory features Not helpful.

Management Genetic counselling, but the variable expression of the disease can give rise to difficulties.

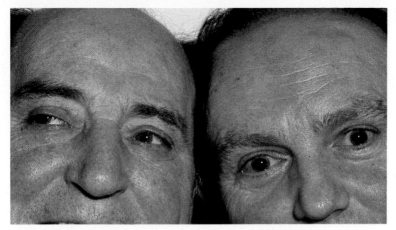

Fig. 213 Osteogenesis imperfecta. Patient with blue sclerae (*right*); control (*left*).

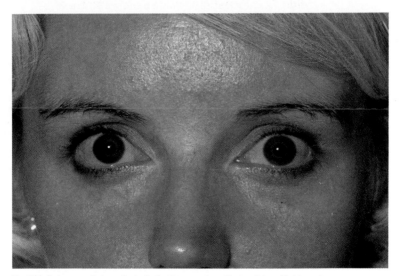

Fig. 214 Osteogenesis imperfecta. Patient's asymptomatic daughter with blue sclerae.

43 / Some other metabolic bone diseases

Diaphyseal aclasis

This is one of the most common inherited skeletal disorders. Multiple bone swellings appear in infancy and increase in number and size until growth stops. The ends of the long bones (Fig. 215), the pelvis and shoulder girdle are most commonly involved. The lesions may be painful or 'silent'. Infrequently, severe deformity and diminution of stature may develop. The most important complication is malignant degeneration.

Albright's syndrome

Named after F. Albright (born 1900) and also termed polyostotic fibrous dysplasia, this disorder is characterized by widespread and often unilateral bone disease, unilateral pigmentation and (in females) precocious puberty. Thyrotoxicosis, acromegaly and Cushing's syndrome may also be associated for reasons yet obscure. The commonest form is the monostotic type, often in the upper end of the femur. The cystic bone changes, which vary in shape and size (Fig. 216), may be extensive and progressive in the polyostotic type. The 'shepherd's crook' deformity of the femur (not shown here) is characteristic. Treatment has included calcitonin (with little success) and orthopaedic correction of deformities.

Synovial osteochondromatosis

This is a condition which is often confused terminologically with osteochondromatosis (previous term for both diaphyseal aclasis and Ollier's disease). It is associated with the formation of cartilaginous plaques within the synovium. By metaplasia these may ossify (Fig. 217). Clinical problems are associated with effusion, 'locking' and premature OA. Treatment is surgical removal of loose bodies or synovectomy.

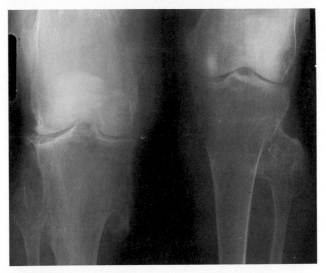

Fig. 215 Diaphyseal aclasis. Massive exostoses at muscle attachments of both knee joints.

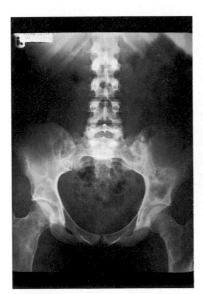

Fig. 216 Albright's syndrome. Cysts in pelvis and femur. Pseudofracture in left femoral neck.

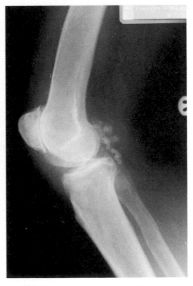

Fig. 217 Synovial osteochondromatosis. Multiple intrasynovial ossified bodies at back of knee joint.

44 / Juvenile chronic arthritis (JCA)

Definition A group of diseases of uncertain aetiology, each of which (by definition) begins before age 16. Although variously labelled 'juvenile rheumatoid arthritis' and 'Still's disease' (after G. F. Still, 1868–1941) in the past, it is now evident that several distinct syndromes are involved.

Prevalence Details not yet known, but the condition is rare. There are probably about 5 000 cases in the UK, i.e. approximately 1:10 000. F:M = 1.7–3.2:1.

Aetiology Probably varies according to type of disease; e.g. juvenile RA probably has different aetiology from juvenile spondarthritis. A varying blend of factors (genetic, environmental and immunological) is likely to be involved.

Clinical and radiological features Clinical types are as follows:

- *Systemic.* Age of onset 1–3 yr. High swinging fever, lymphadenopathy, hepatosplenomegaly, pericarditis and pleurisy are seen. Seronegative for rheumatoid factor.
- *Polyarticular seronegative.* Younger girls.
- *Polyarticular seropositive.* Older girls. Antinuclear factor is positive in 75%.
- *Pauciarticular* (2 types).
  1. Girls under 5 yr. *Chronic* iridocyclitis affects about 5%.
  2. Older boys. Associated with sacroiliitis, HLA-B27 and *acute* iridocyclitis

Both 1 and 2 are seronegative. Other types are seen less often. They may be associated with psoriasis, Reiter's disease, or inflammatory bowel disease; or one of the collagen disorders. (These may or may not be related to one of the 'established' groups.)

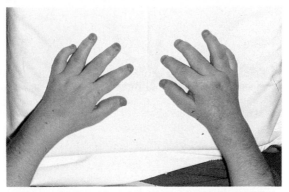

Fig. 218 JCA. Brachydactyly associated with IP and MCP joint arthritis.

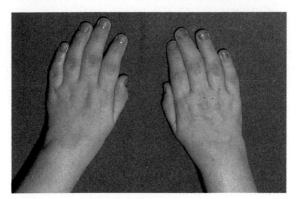

Fig. 219 JCA. Radial deviation at PIP joints.

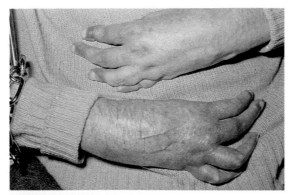

Fig. 220 JCA. Ankylosis and severe deformity with radial deviation (adult).

Clinical and radiological features (contd)

Some characteristic clinical features of the hand arthritis are shown on page 136. Brachydactyly due to metacarpal shortening (Fig. 218), *radial* deviation of fingers (Fig. 219) and ankylosis (Fig. 220) are fairly typical of juvenile, as opposed to adult, rheumatoid arthritis. In addition to involvement of knuckle joints and wrists (and counterpart joints in the feet), other joints may also be involved. In fact no joint is exempt. The knees are commonly affected: Figure 221 demonstrates advanced knee arthritis with valgus deformity (probably aggravated by obesity) and Figure 222 shows severe fixed flexion deformity. (Medical treatment was effective in reducing the latter but not the former.) More often, however, the knee arthritis is no more than a recurring synovitis with effusion, settling over a few years with little residual damage or deformity.

The temporomandibular joints (TMJs) may become arthritic, and dental hygiene may become a problem due to inability to open the mouth sufficiently (Fig. 223). Another repercussion of jaw joint disease is hypoplasia of the mandible. This gives rise to micrognathos (brachygnathism or receding chin), variously termed bird, shrew or mouse facies (Fig. 224). This appearance has been reported in up to 30% of patients. Other growth disturbances due to inhibition or overgrowth of bones will be mentioned overleaf (see 'Management').

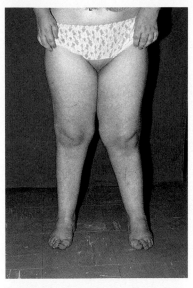

Fig. 221 JCA. Valgus deformity of knees. Note hands and feet also involved.

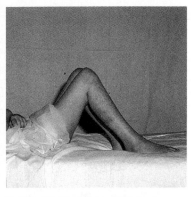

Fig. 222 JCA. Fixed flexion deformity of knees.

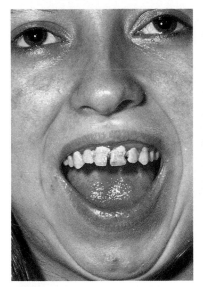

Fig. 223 JCA. Severe dental caries. TMJ involvement.

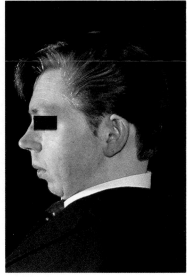

Fig. 224 JCA. Micrognathos ('shrew facies'). TMJs involved.

Clinical and radiological features (contd)

A characteristic feature of some patients with JCA, suggesting a link with the spondarthritides, is sacroiliitis and even fully developed ankylosing spondylitis (Fig. 225). Cervical spine involvement (with fusion) may be particularly troublesome. This illustration, which also shows hip joint fusion, serves to emphasise the strong ankylosing diathesis in peripheral as well as in spinal joints in some juvenile patients. In addition to the non-articular features already mentioned, the rash (Fig. 226) of JCA deserves special mention. This affects about 45% of patients and consists of patches of erythema on the trunk and limbs, often seen towards the end of the day and made prominent by a hot bath. In most patients it is not itchy, but if pruritus is present, it is intense. The rash often shows perimacular blanching ('haloes'), and the Koebner phenomenon may be prominent.

Other associated features, taking JCA as a whole, are fever (20%), splenomegaly (35%), lymphadenopathy (45%); pericarditis (10%), iritis (10%), nodules (5%) and, less commonly, abdominal pain due to mesenteric adenitis or peritonitis. Various CNS effects (drowsiness, irritability, fits, and meningism) are seen in the acute stage.

Laboratory features

See under sub-types (p. 135). In addition, leucocytosis is common in systemic disease.

Management

General principles—drugs, remedial therapy, surgery—are as for adult inflammatory arthritides, with the following exceptions:
- If rest is required, be watchful for development of joint fusion.
- Regular slit-lamp examination for iritis.
- Ensure continued education.
- Avoid contact sports.
- When possible, *avoid systemic corticosteroids* as these may aggravate the natural tendency of the disease to cause growth stunting (Fig. 227).

If necessary use alternate-day steroids or ACTH.

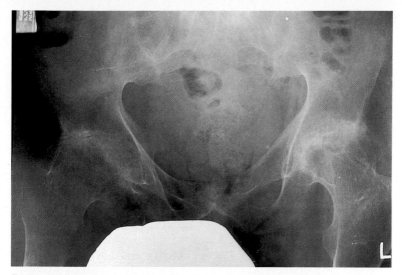

Fig. 225 JCA. Ankylosed sacroiliac joints, hip arthritis and symphyseal changes.

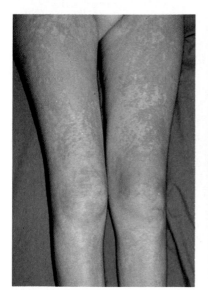

Fig. 226 JCA. Macular erythema.

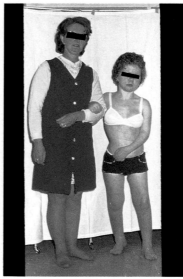

Fig. 227 JCA. Patient with stunted growth (on steroids) standing next to her mother. [Courtesy North-Holland]

45 / Rheumatic fever and rheumatic heart disease

Definition An acute febrile illness, characterized by arthritis, carditis and chorea following streptococcal infection.

Prevalence Now much less frequent and less severe in UK, but still common in some parts of the world. M = F. Peak age of onset: 5–15 yr. The condition is rare below age 3 yr and above 20 yr.

Aetiology Hypersensivity to group-A haemolytic streptococcus. Lesions are probably due to antigen–antibody immune complexes. Predisposing factors include social class (overcrowding), age (children) and slight familial influence.

Clinical features History of sore throat 1–3 weeks before polyarthritis in most patients. The disorder has an acute onset, the main features being arthritis, fever, night sweats, recurrent epistaxis and abdominal pain. The joint disorder is a migratory polyarthritis affecting mainly large joints (knees and ankles commonest). Less commonly other joints may be involved (Fig. 228). Arthritis settles without residua. About 40% develop carditis and a proportion ultimately develop chronic heart disease due to valvular scarring (Fig. 229). Subcutaneous nodules occur in 10%, chorea in 10%, and erythema marginatum in 5%.

Radiological features The joints are normal. Chest X-ray shows cardiac and pulmonary features, especially in chronic rheumatic heart disease with 'decompensation' (Fig. 230).

Laboratory features These include raised ESR; positive throat swab in 25%; ASO titre raised in 75%; raised LDH with carditis; abnormal ECG—conduction defects, signs of pericarditis or myocarditis.

Management
- Rest.
- Aspirin.
- Penicillin in acute phase.
- Treatment of cardiac complications. (Note heart surgery scar in Fig. 229.)

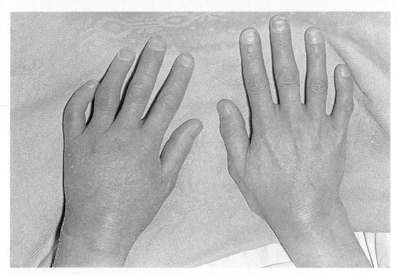

Fig. 228 Rheumatic fever. Acute arthritis of wrist joints and scattered PIP joints.

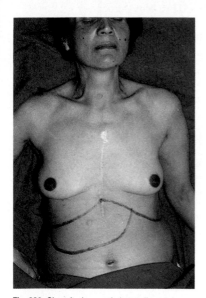

Fig. 229 Chronic rheumatic heart disease. Malar flush, pigmentation, raised JVP, hepatomegaly and cardiac surgery scars.

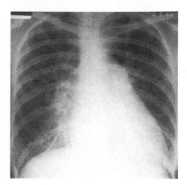

Fig. 230 Mitral stenosis. Straight left heart border, small aortic knuckle, hilar congestion and Kerley's lines.

46 / Henoch–Schönlein purpura and other childhood vasculitides

Henoch–Schönlein purpura

Henoch–Schönlein (or Schönlein–Henoch) purpura is a disorder named after J. L. Schönlein (1793–1864) and E. H. Henoch (1820–1910).

Clinical features The condition is characterized by an exanthem associated with GI manifestations or arthritis, or both. The condition may follow an upper respiratory tract infection which is often streptococcal. The rash, typically found on the buttocks (Fig. 231), is at first urticarial and itchy. Later maculopapular lesions, changing from pink to deep purple, occur. These gradually fade over about 2 weeks. Biopsy of the skin lesions shows characteristic perivascular changes. Arthritis lasts only a few days. Other manifestations tend to last up to 6 weeks but resolve completely, except for the renal disorder which may be more prolonged.

Management Salicylates or other NSAIDs. Not steroids.

Other childhood vaculitides

In addition to Henoch–Schönlein purpura there are many other forms of childhood vasculitis, either occurring as primary diseases or secondary to other systemic disorders. Classification is difficult but follows that proposed for adults, with some exceptions. Figure 232 shows an example of allergic vasculitis which is similar in many respects to Henoch–Schönlein purpura, except that the skin lesions are more varied, more truncal and more prominently urticarial, and GI involvement is less prominent.

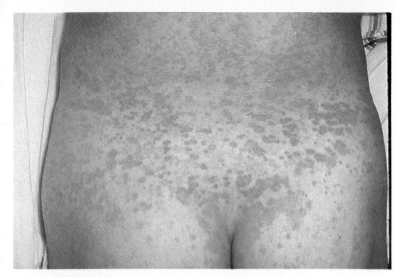

Fig. 231 Henoch–Schönlein purpura. Typical distribution of vasculitic rash.

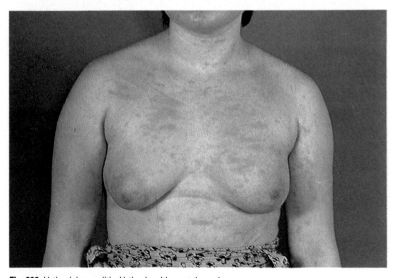

Fig. 232 Urticarial vasculitis. Urticaria with scratch marks.

47 / **Digital contractures/Deformities**

Shoulder–hand syndrome

This is a painful disability of the shoulder appearing before, during, or after pain, swelling and vasomotor changes in the hands and fingers. It may be associated with finger contractures (Fig. 233), and these may evolve into a Dupuytren's-like appearance.

Associated features
These include idiopathic onset (25%); myocardial infarction (20%); cervical spondylosis (20%); trauma (10%); hemiplegia (5%); drugs such as phenobarbitone, isoniazid or ethionamide; malignancy (pulmonary or cerebral); any form of shoulder arthritis; herpes zoster.

Dupuytren's contracture

This is a common disorder in which progressive fibrosis of the palmar fascia causes painless flexion contractures of the fingers.

Prevalence
It affects men more often than women (8:1) and appears after the age of 25 yr. It is occasionally familial and has a significant association with liver disease, especially alcoholic cirrhosis, and epilepsy.

Clinical features
The ring finger is affected first and most prominently, then the little finger, middle finger, index finger and thumb. Puckering of the palmar skin is typical (Fig. 234) and is associated with thickening and sometimes nodules in the palmar fascia. May be associated with knuckle pads or Peyronie's disease. Treated by selective fasciectomy.

Camptodactyly

Implies flexion contracture of PIP joint, typically of the fifth finger (Fig. 235). It may be confused with clinodactyly (see p. 147), and this term is often used synonymously. It may be familial or sporadic.

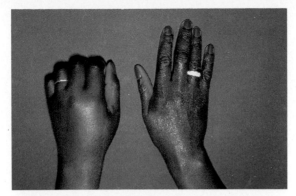

Fig. 233 Shoulder–hand syndrome. Note oedema and digital contracture of left hand.

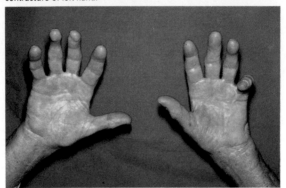

Fig. 234 Dupuytren's contracture. Digital contracture with palmar puckering.

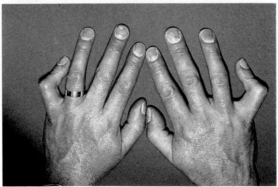

Fig. 235 Camptodactyly. Flexion contracture of both little fingers.

Clinodactyly

Denotes a flexion contracture with radial curvature. This usually affects the PIP joints of the fifth finger (Fig. 236). The condition may occur sporadically or as a familial disorder showing dominant inheritance. Like camptodactyly, it is of little clinical consequence.

Syndactyly

This term refers to bone or soft-tissue union of two or more digits. The extent of the anomaly is variable. Syndactyly is a component of several genetic syndromes. It may exist in isolation either as a genetic or non-genetic entity. In general, the genetic forms are bilateral and fairly symmetrical. Figure 237 shows unilateral (and probably non-genetic) syndactyly.

Polydactyly and polysyndactyly

The presence of an extra digit is termed polydactyly. If digital fusion is also present the term polysyndactyly is used. It may be genetic or non-genetic. Polydactyly is conventionally classified into pre-axial (duplication of thumb or great toe) and postaxial (duplication next to fifth digit). Figure 238 is therefore an example of pre-axial polysyndactyly.

Intrauterine amputation

Intrauterine amputation by amniotic bands is thought to be a common cause of amelia (incidence 1 in 5000–10 000 births). Grooves around limbs or evidence of partial amputation provide additional clues for the action of this process. A typical example of intrauterine amputation is shown in Figure 239.

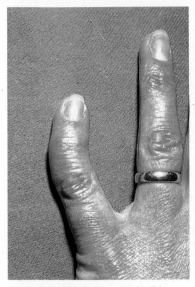

Fig. 236 Clinodactyly. Flexion and radial deviation of little finger.

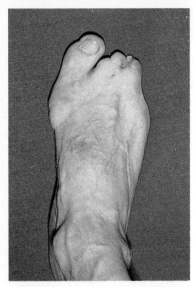

Fig. 237 Syndactyly. Note 'fused' toes and vestigial nail.

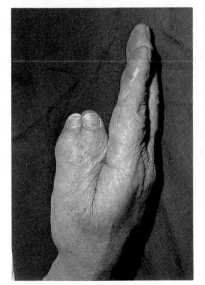

Fig. 238 Polysyndactyly. Double thumbs. (Patient also had nodular RA and pseudoaxanthoma elasticum.)

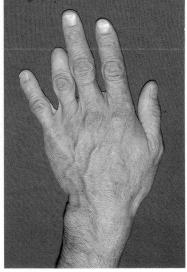

Fig. 239 Intrauterine amputation. Note smooth stump in otherwise normally proportioned finger.

48 / Digital swellings

Knuckle pads

Otherwise known as the knuckle-pad syndrome, knobbly knuckles or Garrod's fatty pads.

Clinical features These appear as fleshy pads over the dorsa of PIP joints (Fig. 240) at any age in either sex. Sometimes painful and tender, and may give rise to suspicion of nodular RA. However, the joints are clinically and radiologically normal. There is often an associated Dupuytren's contracture. Reassurance is the mainstay of therapy.

Neoplastic swellings

Although isolated solid swellings on the fingers are often rheumatoid nodules, Heberden's or Bouchard's nodes, or gouty tophi, occasionally they turn out to be neoplastic. Two examples are shown here (Figs 241 & 242). The ivory osteoma had all the features of a malignant deposit clinically. Remember that renal neoplasms have a particular tendency to metastasize to finger bones.

Cystic swellings

Occasionally Heberden's nodes may appear as cystic swellings. Synovial bulging of PIP joints may also resemble a cyst if localized. The cyst in Figure 243 was an implantation dermoid. Usually there is a history of a penetrating injury. Should be excised if causing inconvenience.

Another cystic swelling in the hand is a ganglion. This is a tense thin-walled cyst that develops over a joint capsule or tendon sheath. Firmness to the point of feeling 'bony' is characteristic of flexor tendon ganglia. A very common site is on the dorsum of the wrist. They may subside spontaneously. If painful, surgical removal is the most effective treatment.

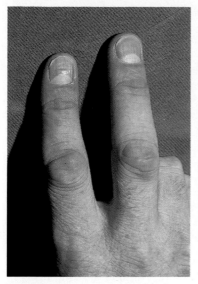

Fig. 240 Knuckle pads. Typical fleshy (and painful) swellings, affecting all fingers.

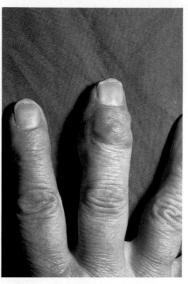

Fig. 241 Synovioma. Biopsy revealed a benign growth.

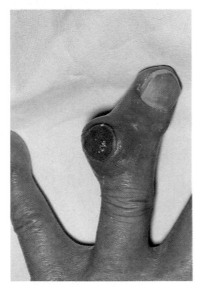

Fig. 242 Ivory osteoma. This ulcerating metastasis-like growth was benign.

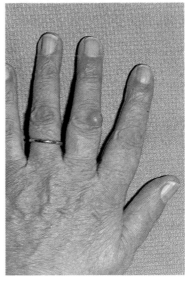

Fig. 243 Implantation dermoid. This cyst appeared without any obvious history of penetrating injury.

Non-steroidal anti-inflammatory drugs (NSAIDs)

When a rash occurs in a patient taking NSAIDs (or any antirheumatic drug for that matter) the question of drug eruption arises. The rash may take many forms, and in many instances mimics that due to a non-iatrogenic cause. The main aid to diagnosis (short of rechallenge) is the knowledge that particular reaction patterns are favoured by certain drugs, and that amongst these some are more common offenders than others. Figure 244 shows aspirin-induced urticaria, the commonest eruption associated with this drug. Other aspirin-induced rashes include angioneurotic oedema, fixed eruptions, erythema multiforme and purpura.

Corticosteroids and corticotrophin

Dermatological manifestation of large doses of corticosteroids or corticotrophin are those associated with hyperactivity of the adrenal cortex: cutaneous atrophy with increased skin fragility, bruising, purpura, striae, local pigmentation, acne, hirsutism and superimposed infections (e.g. buccal candidiasis). More generalized pigmentation may occur with corticotrophin. A typical example of 'steroid skin' is shown in Figure 245—a patient needing long-term corticosteroids for rheumatoid arthritis.

Remission-inducing drugs

Remission-inducing drugs commonly cause rashes. Figure 246 shows a papular erythema associated with penicillamine. Other skin problems due to this drug include purpura, lichenoid and bullous eruptions, and alopecia. Figure 247 typifies the itchy, scaly, delayed dermatitis associated with long-term gold therapy. It may also resemble lichen planus or pityriasis rosea. Acute allergic reactions, including erythema and urticaria, may also occur.

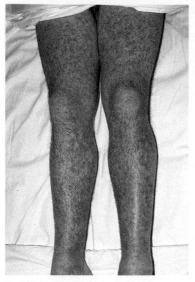

Fig. 244 Aspirin rash. Urticaria. Rapidly subsided on withdrawing drug.

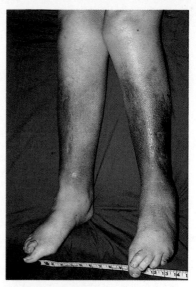

Fig. 245 Steroid skin changes. Dermal atrophy and pigmentation. Scars due to skin tearing. Permanent.

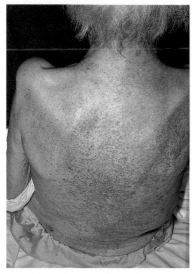

Fig. 246 Penicillamine rash. Papular erythema. Slowly disappeared on withdrawing drug.

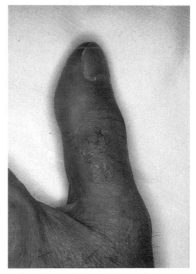

Fig. 247 Gold rash. Scaly, itchy, erythematous patch. Very slowly cleared on withdrawing drug.

50 / **Iatrogenic lesions: other**

Other drug side effects

Some other drug side effects are illustrated here (Figs 248 & 249). Apart from the suspicion that certain drugs are associated with aggravating or even causing peptic ulceration, antirheumatic agents may be associated with other GI effects, e.g. drug-induced dyspepsia by most of them, constipation due to codeine, diarrhoea due to mefenamic acid, aggravation of colitis by indomethacin, precipitation of pancreatitis by corticosteroids and induction of malabsorption by colchicine. The widespread iatrogenic influence of antirheumatic drugs on other systems is too extensive to be included here, but should always be borne in mind.

Problems related to nursing and remedial therapy

Iatrogenic disorders may be encountered during nursing or remedial therapy, e.g. allergy to local agents or dressings (Fig. 250). Other examples of local disease include burns from lamps used in physiotherapy. More serious iatrogenic effects may arise from improper administration of oral or parenteral drugs.

Surgical complications

One of the most feared complications of rheumatological surgery is immediate or delayed infection. Figure 251 shows an infected prosthesis which presented many months after surgery. (This may occur despite the most meticulous technique, including the use of local and systemic antibiotics, and specially designed—laminar flow—operating theatres.)

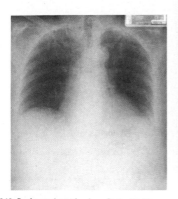

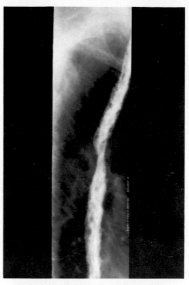

Fig. 248 Perforated peptic ulcer. Patient taking steroids and indomethacin. Note gas under right diaphragm.

Fig. 249 Monilial oesophagitis. Patient taking large doses of antibiotics for septic arthritis.

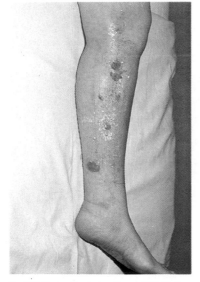

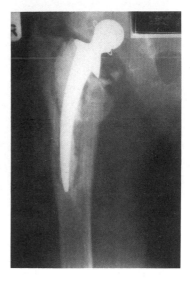

Fig. 250 Zinc oxide plaster allergy. Patient on leg traction for disc prolapse.

Fig. 251 Infected prosthesis. Note lucent zone around prosthesis/cement outline.

Index

Only affected structure tissues receiving important mentions have been indexed. Some important structures (e.g. hands, feet, limbs) occur too often to be indexed. For such structures, only those conditions in which the structure forms part of the name (e.g. finger clubbing, sacroiliitis) have been indexed.